D0582394

Pilates
for
Pregnancy

GENTLE AND EFFECTIVE TECHNIQUES …
FOR BEFORE AND AFTER BIRTH

Anna Selby

Foreword by Clare Fone, MCSP, SRP

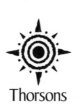

Thorsons

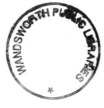
WANDSWORTH PUBLIC LIBRARIES

Thorsons
An Imprint of HarperCollins*Publishers*
77–85 Fulham Palace Road,
Hammersmith, London W6 8JB

The Thorsons website is www.thorsons.com

and *Thorsons*
are trademarks of HarperCollins*Publishers* Limited

First published 2002

1 3 5 7 9 10 8 6 4 2

500 736598
© Anna Selby 2002

Anna Selby asserts the moral right to
be identified as the author of this work

A catalogue record for this book
is available from the British Library

ISBN 0 00 713314 6

Photographs © Guy Hearn

Printed and bound in Great Britain by
Martins the Printers Ltd., Berwick-upon-Tweed

All rights reserved. No part of this publication may be
reproduced, stored in a retrieval system, or transmitted,
in any form or by any means, electronic, mechanical,
photocopying, recording or otherwise, without the prior
permission of the publishers.

Contents

All of the exercises in this book are designed to be suitable for pregnancy or as post-natal exercises. However, it is always advisable to check with your doctor before you begin any course of exercise and particularly so at this time. It is especially important to take care during the first three months of pregnancy, when the risk of miscarriage is at its highest. It is also invaluable to have some lessons with a qualified Pilates teacher. There is nothing like an experienced eye for picking up problems and recommending ways of solving them, or simply for placing you in correct alignment for the exercises. Once you have felt the integrity of your body working as a whole, you will know what to do every time you exercise.

Foreword

When I was asked to write a foreword to a book totally dedicated to Pilates during and after pregnancy, I was delighted to do so. Having had three babies myself – and the last one was 11 pounds 6 ounces – I have personally found Pilates to be a fantastic form of exercise. It is safe, specific and can be performed even with an injury. It is a 'feel good' technique that ties in beautifully with our own treatments as chartered physiotherapists.

As a pregnancy develops and the baby grows bigger, your normal posture changes and a strain is put on joints, muscles and all the soft tissues. Movement becomes more restricted and the blood supply to the tissues is reduced. Normal breathing patterns are disturbed as the internal organs fight for space. The pelvic floor muscles can be weakened during pregnancy, leading to incontinence later. Pilates addresses all of these problems. It mobilizes all your neural tissues, focuses throughout on breathing and incorporates pelvic floor exercises.

Pregnancy is a precious time with your developing baby and it is terribly important to feel good about yourself and your changing body. Exercising the Pilates way will reap rewards both during and after your pregnancy – and will help you to avoid the problems caused by poor posture that, as physiotherapists, we see all the time.

The exercises in this book are very clear, gentle and easy to follow. I defy anyone not to feel good with these programmes for during and after pregnancy.

Clare Fone MCSP, SRP, Cert. Health Ed.
Westminster Physiotherapy Centre

Using this book

Certain exercises have been marked with an icon to indicate that they focus on specific areas of the body.

 During pregnancy, it's vital to strengthen the pelvic floor muscles. Most Pilates exercises have this effect to some degree, but these exercises are particularly effective.

 During the second and especially the third trimesters of pregnancy, many women suffer from Oedema – a swelling in the hands, feet and ankles due to excess fluid. These exercises are recommended for this condition.

What is the Pilates Method?

The Pilates method originated around a hundred years ago near Düsseldorf in Germany, when a frail child called Joseph Pilates took up body-building to increase his strength. At the time he was thought to be prone to tuberculosis, as well as being generally weak and sickly but, so successful was the programme he devised, that by the age of 14, he was posing as a model for anatomical drawings.

He went on to become a keen sportsman – a gymnast, skier, boxer, diver, and even a circus performer. In 1912, Pilates left his native Germany and moved to England where, at the outbreak of the First World War, he was interned as an enemy alien. Pilates used his enforced leisure to develop his method of attaining peak physical fitness.

Pilates called his new system 'muscle contrology', and through it he aimed to bring about the complete co-ordination of body, mind and spirit, working *with* – not on or against – the body's muscles. After the war, he returned briefly to Germany and then moved to New York where his 'contrology' method was an immediate success, particularly with dancers such as Martha Graham and George Balanchine, the founder of the New York City Ballet. Pilates' exercise method remained something of a secret amongst dancers until comparatively recently, when sportsmen, actors and the public began to discover it. The popularity of Pilates has soared over the last few years.

THE ORIGINAL PILATES METHOD

Much of Pilates' early work was based on the rehabilitation of ill or injured people. During his internment, when Pilates worked as a nurse, he had experimented devising an exercise regime by attaching springs to hospital beds, so that patients could begin to work on toning their muscles even before they could get up. Springs used as resistance were the cornerstone of his method and Pilates designed a machine that he called the 'universal reformer', a sliding horizontal bed that can be used with up to four springs, according to the exercise and the strength of the individual. On this machine, one can perform pliés and other exercises without putting any weight on the joints (so beneficial for those with injuries or other joint problems), and against resistance (so that the muscles are worked harder).

Pilates developed several other machines for his New York studio and these have been adapted and used around the world ever since. More recently, the principles of the Pilates method have been adapted for use without machines and this system has become particularly popular. It is this version of Pilates that has been used in this book. It is an especially gentle version, particularly in those exercises recommended for the pregnancy itself; in the post-pregnancy section, the exercises become more strenuous and complex, but build on the same principles that are the foundation of all Pilates work. In fact, because it is so important to understand these basic principles, even if you begin the exercises after you have had your baby, it is still important to go back to the first section of the book and work through this before you go on to the second part.

The Pilates Principles

The Pilates method has changed substantially over the decades but its underlying principles remain the same. One of these is that Pilates is, quite simply, the thinking person's exercise. Unlike the kind of workout that involves jumping around to loud music, where your main priority is to keep up, in Pilates every movement is carefully controlled for maximum effect. To work, it requires concentration. For each and every exercise, there are questions you need to ask yourself. Is the navel drawn towards the spine? Is the heel in the correct position? Is the neck long and aligned with the spine? Is your breathing correct?

In the Pilates method, the placing and movement of every part of your body counts and the body works as an integrated system. The more you use your body correctly during exercise, the more you will use it correctly in everything you do. Your posture improves and the headaches, tight, contracted muscles and tensions that arise from poor posture all fade away.

Interestingly, all this concentration does not leave you mentally drained or exhausted. On the contrary, it is a profoundly relaxing method of exercise and its slow, rhythmic movements are a stress relief in themselves, and leave most people feeling simultaneously calm and energized. This mental relaxation, in turn, helps bring about physical relaxation, as your muscles become less tense.

In the long term, the effect of Pilates on the body is to give your muscles a lengthened, toned shape rather than bulk. Think of a dancer's body, rather than a gym fanatic's. Obviously, in the short term while you are pregnant, your exercising priorities are different: you need to give protection to your back, strengthen the pelvic floor, keep your muscles generally toned and learn to relax both physically and mentally. Pilates will help you to do all of these things and, while your body is in its exceptionally sensitive and perceptive pregnant state, you can assimilate the principles of the method particularly easily.

THE PRINCIPLES

Before you begin the exercises, it is important to understand the theory that underlies the Pilates method. These are the essential principles to bear in mind whenever you exercise:

1. **Concentration:** As I have already said, concentration is fundamental to this way of exercising. This is not only because it is important that every part of your body is moving or positioned correctly – a part of

a synchronized whole. It is also because, when you concentrate on your body in this way, it actually leads your mind away from any immediate concerns or anxieties, and is profoundly relaxing.

2. **The breath:** The way you breathe is vitally important within the Pilates method. There are two breathing exercises in the warm-up to ensure that you are breathing correctly and, even if you feel that this is obvious, they really do help to make you breathe deeply, rhythmically and to your full capacity. The other point to remember is *when* you breathe: in Pilates exercises, you breathe out with the effort. This helps you to relax into a movement. If you breathe in for the effort of an exercise, you will automatically tense up.

3. **The 'girdle of strength':** According to Joseph Pilates, the girdle of strength was essential for all exercise. This 'girdle' incorporates three main areas – the back, the abdomen and the buttocks. The upper back can be a major seat of tension but when you learn to move the arms correctly (from the middle of the back rather than the shoulders), this tension will disappear. Nearly every exercise in this book begins by drawing the navel gently towards the spine. This both strengthens the transverse abdominal muscles so that you will – eventually! – regain a flat stomach, and protects the back against undue strain during the exercise. (In contrast, normal aerobic exercises do not concentrate on the transverse abdominal muscles, and so a potbelly remains!) The third element in this girdle of strength is the buttock muscles. By engaging and squeezing these during the exercises, you not only tone the muscles themselves you also bring the body into perfect alignment, improving the posture and protecting the back from strain or injury.

4. **Flowing movements:** Unlike many forms of exercise, Pilates is not based on sudden, jerky movements. Instead, one position flows as slowly and naturally as possible into the next. You move rhythmically, your pace set by your own breathing and this warms the muscles and makes them lengthen out rather than bunch and bulk up. Moving slowly also gives you time to become aware of each part of your body so that you perform all the exercises with precision and in a co-ordinated way.

5. **Relaxation:** This is an important element of the method at any time but none more so than during pregnancy. The warm-up exercises that you should do before all of your exercise sessions – both during and after pregnancy – help to reduce and remove the most common areas of tension in the body, slow down the breathing and focus the mind. The relaxation exercises at the end of the session are also important. During pregnancy or when you have broken nights with a new baby, you are often overwhelmed with feelings of tiredness. This final relaxation will help to restore flagging energy levels and, just as crucially, to induce a more tranquil state of mind.

Pilates and Pregnancy

HOW YOUR BODY CHANGES DURING PREGNANCY

Until you have actually been pregnant, it is hard to imagine how many changes your body can go through in such a short time. Many women notice changes even before their first missed period – sore or enlarged breasts, for instance, or feelings of nausea are not uncommon. These changes and the greater ones to come are triggered by a massive increase of hormones during pregnancy.

The role of the hormones is to create the right conditions for maintaining your pregnancy and for nourishing your baby and they are released from the moment your baby has implanted in your womb. The main hormones involved are oestrogen and progesterone and they increase to around 100 times higher than their normal level during your pregnancy, dropping back to the usual levels immediately after the birth. One of the effects of these hormones is to make your muscles soften and relax to allow room for your baby to grow inside you.

A third hormone, relaxin, is also released and, as its name suggests, its effect, too, is to relax the body. This hormone affects the ligaments – the connective tissue between the bones – so that the pelvis can soften and expand in preparation for the birth. Interestingly, endorphins – the body's natural feel-good hormones – also increase during pregnancy and this may account for the 'glow' of pregnancy, especially from the second trimester (three-month period) onwards, when you often feel particularly calm and content.

All of these hormonal changes within the body are clearly a preparation for pregnancy and birth but they have other effects, too, that need to be considered when it comes to your exercise routine. Because you have around nine extra pints of blood by the end of your pregnancy, your heart has to work much harder to pump it all around your body. Pilates exercises do not raise the heart rate, and if you are doing extra cardiovascular work, you should be careful not to raise your heart rate too high, especially as the foetal heart rate is already substantially higher than an adult's. Pilates, yoga and gentle swimming and walking are all ideal forms of exercise for this reason.

The increase in hormones that relax the ligaments and muscles means you are much more supple than usual. You become looser very quickly and this mobility will be very noticeable during exercise, particularly in forms like yoga and Pilates where stretching plays a major part. The drawback to this is that your joints can become unstable and, if you do not keep your abdominal muscles toned, the back in particular may be at risk of strain. The roll-downs (*see page* 24) and posture checks (*see page* 16) are all important to prevent damage to your back, especially in later pregnancy when the weight of the baby changes your centre of gravity and tends to induce a 'sway back' in your stance.

Your breasts also enlarge rapidly with the pregnancy from its earliest days. Their extra weight can put a strain on the neck, shoulders and upper back, as well as undermining your posture by rounding your shoulders. During pregnancy, you need to do plenty of exercises that release tension in this area and also increase mobility and postural awareness. It is vital to buy a well-fitting bra that will give you support at each stage of your pregnancy. Always go to a store where they have a fitting service.

The extra blood in your body is not the only increased fluid of pregnancy. The lymphatic fluid – essentially, your body's waste disposal system – the amniotic fluid that surrounds your baby, and the fluid to all of your bodily tissues increase too. Regular exercise helps to keep this fluid moving and prevent oedema (water retention and swelling) and drinking plenty of water has a similar effect – surprising as it may seem. Drinking plenty of water is also very important after the birth, especially when breastfeeding, and generally throughout your life, as dehydration is now thought to be an underlying factor in many ailments.

The relaxing effect of the hormones causes the walls of your blood vessels to relax, too, and this can lead to varicose veins as well as varicosities in the vulva or anus (haemorrhoids or piles). Exercise generally, and pelvic floor exercises in particular, will help to reduce the risk.

The digestive system is also affected by pregnancy. One of the first signs of pregnancy is morning sickness and this can take the form of feelings of nausea or actual vomiting. This usually disappears after the third month of pregnancy. Digestion slows down during pregnancy and this can result in heartburn or constipation. Exercise helps your metabolism speed up generally and, again, reduces these risks.

After the birth of your baby, your body starts to return to its pre-pregnant state, reducing hormonal output and fluid balance immediately. Breast-feeding will speed up this process. It may feel that you have a long way to go, especially if you were expecting to regain a flat abdomen straightaway. You can get your body back in shape, but take care not to rush things at the start. Give yourself time to recover, rest and relax into your new role.

EXERCISE DURING PREGNANCY

Exercise is important for you during your pregnancy on a number of levels – but it is vital that it is the right sort of exercise. Pregnancy is a time to focus on stretching, relaxing and gentle toning, rather than vigorous exercise aimed at building muscle and stamina. If you are already very fit, you may want or be able to keep up your normal exercise routine, just adapting it to take your new condition into account. Pregnancy is *not*, though, a time to try to *get* fit – leave demanding exercise regimes until some time after the birth.

During the first trimester strenuous exercise should be avoided by all pregnant women, because this is the period when miscarriage is most likely. At this time, it is better to concentrate on improving your posture, strengthening the pelvic floor, relaxation and breathing. Pregnancy often gives you a heightened perception of your own body and so it is an ideal time to learn Pilates technique, emphasizing as it does concentrated, aware exercise. Many women feel extremely tired during the first three months of pregnancy, and some feelings of nausea are likely – and these can occur at any time, not just in the mornings. It is important to rest whenever you feel the need and you can go through the relaxation sequence (*see page* 45) whenever you feel stressed or tired.

The second trimester, or mid-period of your pregnancy, is very different from the first. All signs of nausea usually disappear, together with the worst of the tiredness as your body settles into its pregnant state. You often feel extremely well both physically and emotionally. This is the time when your pregnancy becomes more visible to the outside world and, as your shape changes, it is important to exercise in the correct way to protect against strain and injury, to boost the circulation of both blood and lymph, to keep muscles toned and for your own sense of well-being.

The final trimester is when many women feel their extra weight to be an almost unbearable burden and the final weeks seem to drag. Exercise is of great benefit now, especially in reducing oedema and correcting postural imbalances caused by the extra weight of the breasts and the baby. Relaxation and breathing techniques also enable you to experience a profound rest that is often very welcome at a time when your sleep patterns are disrupted. Lying on your back can be quite uncomfortable now – if so, you should avoid any exercises in this position and concentrate on those that are more comfortable. Kneeling on all fours is a good position in late pregnancy both for exercising and relaxing, as it takes the weight of the baby off the spine.

After the birth of your baby, you will naturally want to get back in shape. However, it is important not to rush back into a vigorous exercise regime. You will have your final post-natal check-up six weeks after the birth and until you have that all-clear, confine your routine to pelvic floor exercises. If you have had a Caesarean section, you will need to wait a good deal longer – up to six months, but check with your doctor. Take it slowly whatever type of birth you have had. Your breasts will still be bigger and heavier than usual while you are breastfeeding and the muscles and ligaments will remain soft – and so easy to strain – for some time to come. Therefore it is important not to – literally – overstretch yourself too soon. The sections in the second, post-pregnancy part of the book are divided into three-month periods. However, these are as a guide only. Progress at your own speed, err on the side of caution and make sure you can do all the exercises in each section comfortably before you move on.

THE IMPORTANCE OF POSTURE

Posture is an old-fashioned word but it is of the utmost importance to all of us, and at no time is this more true than during pregnancy. One of the fundamentals of the Pilates technique is establishing good posture, both in terms of how you perform the exercises and how this is carried over into the way you use your body in your everyday life. Good posture prevents all manner of strains, aches and pains, headaches and injuries. It also instantly improves the way you look. And by ensuring that your posture is good all the time – not just when you are exercising – every movement you make becomes a way of toning and strengthening the body. Many years ago, I had my first Pilates lessons with Dreas Reyneke in London, and they were a re-education in how I used my body. I can clearly remember leaving after the third lesson and realizing I was walking in a completely new way that made me feel wonderful, as if I had suddenly connected in some fundamental way with my body.

Even if you have good posture to start with, pregnancy can be a time when it deteriorates. This is particularly true as the pregnancy advances and the weight of the baby moves your centre of gravity forwards, often resulting in an extreme hollowing in the lower back. This in turn can result in the lower back pain so common in pregnancy, as well as serious, long-term back problems. At the same time, the increased weight of the breasts can pull the shoulders forwards and distort the neck and the way the head is held. Your spine can end up in an exaggerated S shape and when this happens, pains and strains are not far behind.

Maintaining a good posture during, and after, pregnancy brings so many benefits:
1. It releases muscle tension.
2. It improves the blood supply to all tissues and organs.
3. It improves the functioning of the autonomic nervous system, which in turn improves the functioning of the reproductive organs.
4. It reduces the strain on your muscles, joints and ligaments.

Pilates exercises are designed to make you aware of every part of your body so that you move it in perfect alignment. Ultimately, these exercises will deliver a graceful, elongated body – but you must do them correctly, slowly and with concentration, and that is why you should begin every exercise session you do by checking and aligning your posture with the exercises below. If you are not in the correct position during an exercise, you will not get the full benefits from Pilates, which is why you should, ideally, arrange for a few individual sessions with a Pilates instructor, or a chartered physiotherapist with a good awareness of muscle imbalance, if you can.

STANDING POSTURE

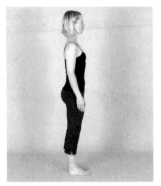

Ideally, you should set up two full-length mirrors for this, so that you can check both the front and side view of your posture. Illustrated here is the posture you should aim for both when you are exercising and in your everyday life. Pilates is all about using the body correctly all of the time. When you stand correctly, you are much more likely to be using the right muscles to make every movement, whether that happens to be a Pilates exercise or when you are simply reaching for a high shelf. During pregnancy, your centre of gravity moves so it is more important than ever to keep the right alignment in order to avoid back ache, tension in the shoulders and neck, headache and many other related problems. Just because you are not moving during this exercise, it does not mean that none of your muscles is working – check that each part of your body is in the right alignment and working correctly.

First Trimester

Head and neck
The head should sit relaxed and balanced on the top of the spine with the neck long and in line with the spine. If you tip your chin up or jut it out, you will pull the neck out of alignment with the spine and this distortion will have serious consequences for your posture, creating tension in several muscle groups and, quite possibly, headaches. The chin should be tipped very slightly down to lengthen the back of the neck, and you should feel as if the top of your head is attached to a piece of string pulling you up and lengthening you out.

Shoulders and arms
The shoulders and upper back often hold a great deal of the body's tension, much of it due to incorrect posture. All arm movement should originate in the muscles of the middle back beneath the shoulder blades and the shoulders themselves should not lift up just because the arms do. Lift the shoulders up to your ears and just let them drop down into a relaxed position – this is where they should be all of the time. The arms should hang comfortably by your sides, without tension. Looking straight at the mirror, check that the shoulders are at an even height – sometimes one is tensed and held higher than the other, especially if you always carry a bag on the same side. Turn sideways to the mirror and check that the shoulders are neither pulled back, which distorts the neck, nor slouched forward.

Back and stomach

Stand sideways on to the mirror to check your back. Let your spine lengthen out, the tailbone dropping towards the floor. Draw the navel gently towards the spine and gently pull up the pelvic floor muscles, so that you do not overarch in the small of the back and your bottom does not stick out. Using these muscles protects the back from strain and is part of the Pilates 'girdle of strength'.

Buttocks

When your navel and back are in the correct placement, your pelvis will tilt very slightly upwards. If you gently squeeze the lowest muscles in the buttocks, this will help you keep the right alignment.

Legs and feet

Your feet should be a hip-width apart, with the toes facing forwards, not turned out. The legs should feel long and pulled up without overextending the knees, pushing them too far back. Feel the weight evenly distributed between both feet.

Second and Third Trimesters

During the later months of your pregnancy, you are aiming at essentially the same posture as above, but your body is subject to different pressures and an altered centre of gravity. The main effect will be on the curvature of your spine when the weight of the baby can move your centre of gravity further forwards, hollowing out the lower back. This makes the strength of the muscles that draw your navel back towards the spine more important than ever, as they will protect you from the lower back pain that is so common in late pregnancy.

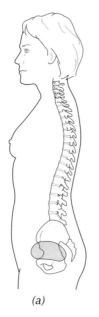

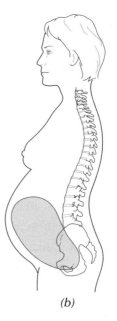

(a)

Not pregnant

(b)

Pregnant.
The spinal curves
are exaggerated as
the weight of the
uterus increases.

In Pilates technique, the elongation of the spine helps to prevent exaggerating the spinal curvature during pregnancy. It also helps the ribcage to expand, improving your breathing. The slight pelvic tilt in a good postural position holds your baby securely from below and helps you to strengthen your pelvic floor muscles at the same time.

SITTING POSTURE

When you are sitting down, especially during the later months of the pregnancy, make sure your back is supported and your feet are flat on the floor. Let the weight drop down into the pelvis and lengthen the spine, relaxing the shoulders, but trying not to slouch. Remember not to cross your legs, as this blocks your circulation.

When you get up from a chair, the important thing to remember is to protect your back. It is all too easy when pregnancy has brought your centre of gravity forwards for you to hollow in the back when you start to get up. To avoid this, place the feet at least a hip-width apart, one around six inches in front of the other. Lean forwards over your legs and then rise up using the muscles in the thighs and buttocks, not the back.

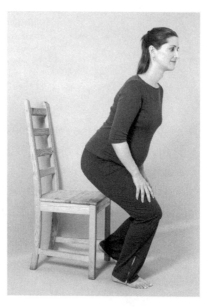

Exercising While Pregnant

Exercising While Pregnant

part
one

4

The Warm-Up

This section is the first stage of *each* exercise session, from the first stages of pregnancy right through to six months after the birth (and ever after!). A Pilates warm-up is very different from others you may have experienced. Rather than working to warm up the muscles and increase the heart rate, in Pilates your focus is on posture and alignment, locating and isolating the areas you will be using. These exercises also relax you and help to bring your focus on to your body, relieving your mind of everyday concerns. Do them slowly and carefully.

Roll Down Against Wall

This exercise mobilizes and places the spine in its correct alignment. This and the following exercise are ideal warm-ups at every stage of your pregnancy and after the birth.

If you feel dizzy at any point during this exercise, stop immediately.

1. Stand 6–8 inches away from a wall with your knees slightly bent and feet hip-width apart, toes facing forwards. Measure out the length of your spine against the wall, with the head held high on a long neck and the shoulders relaxed. Your arms hang comfortably at your sides. Draw your navel gently to the spine.

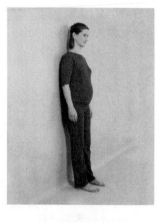

2. Breathe in and, as you breathe out, pull up the muscles of the pelvic floor and drop your chin to your chest, feeling the stretch all the way through the neck and upper back. As you begin to mobilize the spine, the arms will move naturally – just let them hang, don't try to place them.

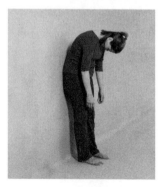

3. Let the curve deepen so that your back peels away from the wall in a long curve, head and arms hanging down until only the buttocks are touching the wall. Breathe naturally for a few moments as your body hangs upside down and relaxes into the stretch.

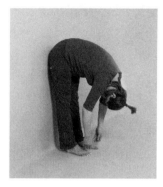

4. On the next out-breath, check that your navel is still drawn towards the spine and the pelvic floor muscles are pulled up and rotate from the pelvis to bring yourself back to a standing position, feeling your back touch the wall vertebra by vertebra. As your back unrolls, feel your shoulders drop down naturally. The head comes in line with the spine, last of all. Check that your back is long, your neck and shoulders are relaxed and your 'girdle of strength' is working. Repeat the whole exercise three times.

Slide Down Wall

This is another postural exercise. It lengthens the spine, teaches correct alignment and works the thigh muscles.

1. Stand near a wall, as you did in the previous exercise. Measure out the length of your spine against the wall, with the head held high on a long neck and shoulders relaxed. Your arms should hang comfortably at your sides. Draw your navel gently to the spine.

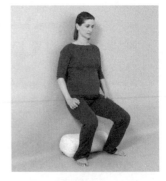

2. Breathe in and, as you breathe out, pull up the pelvic floor muscles and bend your knees more deeply so that your back starts to slide down the wall. Take care not to go down any further than your thighs are able to support your weight without lifting you heels off the floor or letting any part of your back come away from the wall. In the later stages of pregnancy, you may want to put a large cushion on the floor, so you can rest in this position.

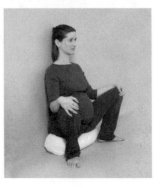

3. Breathe in and slide back up. Repeat up to 5 times.

5

First Trimester

During the first trimester it is best to keep strenuous exercise to a minimum, as this is the time when the risk of miscarriage is at its highest. It is also a time when many women feel unbelievably tired and nauseous – so not particularly inclined to exercise much anyway. Instead, as early pregnancy makes you increasingly aware and intuitive about your body, this is a good time to focus on your posture. Getting this right now ensures that your practice throughout your pregnancy and beyond will have the right foundation. One series of exercises that are really important now, though, are the pelvic floor exercises. Do these as often as possible, not just during an exercise session – standing waiting for a bus will do just as well! The other exercises for this trimester include gentle stretching, especially to release tension from the upper body, breathing and relaxation techniques.

Pelvic Floor Exercises

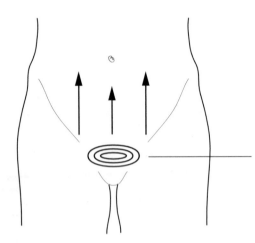

Pelvic Floor Muscle Group

You can exercise this important muscle group by contracting your pelvic floor. Imagine you are 'lifting' the pelvic floor upwards.

If you do nothing else during your pregnancy – do these exercises! The importance of strengthening your pelvic floor muscles now just cannot be overstated. These muscles support everything that is above them and, during pregnancy, your baby and the extra weight of the uterus increase their load considerably. Having strong pelvic floor muscles will help you during the birth and they are less likely to be damaged during labour. In the long term, weak pelvic floor muscles can lead to incontinence, haemorrhoids and even prolapse of the uterus, so it is worth strengthening them now.

First of all, you need to locate your pelvic floor muscles. Because they are internal, many people are not even aware of them and this is particularly the case if the muscles themselves are weak. If you are not sure where they are, perhaps the easiest way to find them is by stopping and starting the flow of urine in midstream. These are the muscles that you contract and release in the following exercises.

You can do these exercises anywhere – standing up or sitting down. Squatting on your heels with your knees apart is a good way of testing the muscles, as they need to work harder in order to contract fully. If you have haemorrhoids or varicose veins, however, simply sit on a chair with your feet flat on the floor instead. You can repeat them as many times and as often as you like, and you can also include them in any exercises where you 'draw the navel to the spine' – when you can pull up the pelvic floor muscles at the same time.

1. **Contract and release**
    Slowly contract your pelvic floor muscles in a long upward movement towards the uterus. Your body should not move outwardly as you do this and your abdomen and buttocks should remain relaxed. Hold and then slowly release. Work towards holding them for a longer count each time, working up to 10.

2. **The lift**
    Contract your pelvic floor muscles in the same way as in the previous exercises but this time pause three times during the upward movement like a lift stopping on every floor. Hold at the top and release, stage by stage, on the way down.

3. **Pulses**
    Contract all the pelvic floor muscles in one go and then release rapidly. Do this repeatedly in time with your pulse.

Breathing Exercises

In Pilates exercises, you use the breath in a very specific way. For the most part, all movement and effort takes place on the out-breath, while on the in-breath you are stretching, preparing or relaxing. This is very different from many forms of exercise where the effort is made on the in-breath – think of the weightlifter's grunted inhalation. Breathing in on the effort results in tension and bunching in the muscles, whereas when you make the effort on the out-breath, in the Pilates way, you elongate the muscles.

Many of us breathe shallowly and rapidly, our lungs far from reaching their potential to fill completely. When you breathe deeply, oxygen circulates more efficiently through the body, nourishing both you and your baby. Slow breathing is both energizing and relaxing, and at the end of this section there are exercises using the breath as an aid to relaxation. The breathing exercises that follow here show you how to breathe fully and expansively in the deep, rhythmic way that shapes all of the exercises to come.

1. **Awareness of the abdomen**

    Lie on your back with a small cushion underneath your head and your feet up on a chair so that your knees form a right angle. Put a small cushion or rolled-up towel between your knees and keep it in place throughout. Check that your back is long and straight and that there is no tension in the neck or shoulders. Place your hands on the abdomen so that your middle fingers are barely touching. As you breathe in, the inhalation should reach all the way down to the abdomen and part the fingers. As you breathe out, the fingers should meet again. Try not to exaggerate this movement and do not push the abdomen out or arch in the back. Just try to feel the breath filling the body. Repeat for 10 breaths.

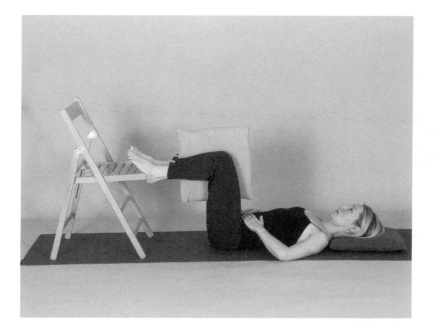

2. **Awareness of the ribs**

Sit on a ball or chair with your feet firmly on the floor, a hip-width apart, toes pointing forwards. Feel your back long and straight with no tension in the neck or shoulders. Wrap a long scarf around your back at rib level, cross it at the front and hold one end in each hand, keeping the scarf taut but not tight throughout. Breathe in deeply – checking that your shoulders do not rise when you do so – and feel your ribs expanding so that you have to release the scarf slightly. Breathe out and feel the ribs contract. Repeat for 10 breaths.

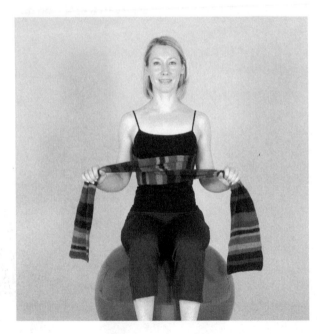

Head Rolls and Tilts

Many people store tension in their shoulders and necks, so these exercises and those that follow aim to release that tension and put the spine in proper alignment. Early pregnancy is a good time to start these exercises if you haven't done them before. If you can break these kinds of bad habits now and find your true, elongated posture, you will reap great rewards in terms of how you feel later in the pregnancy.

1. Sit with your feet flat on the floor with a long, straight back. Draw the navel gently to the spine and pull up the pelvic floor. Check there is no tension in the shoulders, neck or face – particularly the jaw, forehead and around the eyes. Take a few long, deep breaths and let yourself relax.

2. Drop your chin down to your chest, without moving or tensing the shoulders. Roll the head around towards the right until your ear is above the shoulder. Slowly roll back to the centre and then continue to the left. Repeat 4–5 times on each side, checking each time that there is no tension or movement in the shoulders. Return to the central position and lift the head.

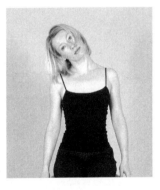

3. Now turn the head to look over your right shoulder. Keep the back of the neck long and released, and the chin slightly tucked in. Return to the centre and turn to the left. Repeat 4–5 times on each side.

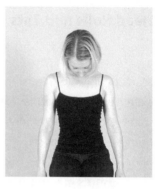

Shoulder Lifts and Circles

These exercises help to release the upper body, particularly the neck, shoulders and back. Before you begin, take time to check the body is alert but relaxed.

Sit as in the previous exercise, with a long straight spine. Take a few long, deep breaths and let yourself completely relax. Tilt your chin down slightly and feel that your neck is in line with your spine.

1. Lift your shoulders up as high as you can towards your ears, letting your arms hang loosely at your sides. Let them drop down heavily, rather than placing them. Repeat 5 times. Now lift just the right shoulder 5 times, then repeat the exercise on the left.

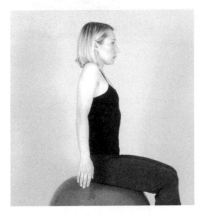 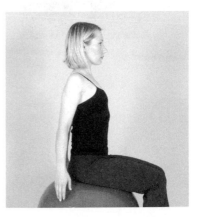

2. Draw the shoulders forwards so that you close up the front of the chest and, in a long, slow movement circle them up towards the ears and then to the back so that you squeeze the shoulder blades together. If you feel any tension in the neck, drop the head forwards slightly. Repeat 5 times then reverse the direction so that you start at the back and circle towards the front.

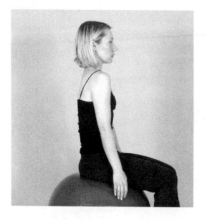 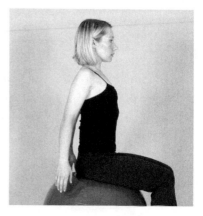

Arm Stretches

These stretches have a double function. They both tone the arms and bring awareness of how you should move them, particularly where the movement originates. When you move your arms from the shoulder blades rather than by lifting the shoulders themselves, your posture improves and you are much less likely to experience tension in the back and neck. The best way to check you are moving correctly is to do this exercise in front of a mirror. If you find the first exercise too easy, hold a food can in each hand as a homemade weight.

1. Sit on a ball or chair with your feet flat on the floor with a long, straight back. Draw the navel gently to the spine and pull up the pelvic floor. Check there is no tension in the shoulders, neck or face – particularly the jaw, forehead and around the eyes. Take a few long, deep breaths and let yourself relax.

2. Drop your arms down to your sides and loosely clench your fists. Breathe in and, as you breathe out, slowly lift the arms straight up to the sides so they are just below shoulder level. The arms should feel both a lift and a stretch and the shoulders should remain completely still. Repeat 5–10 times slowly.

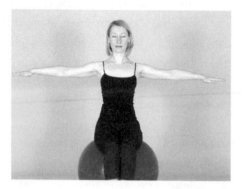

3. Drop your arms down to your sides and stretch your fingers. Breathe in and, as you breathe out, slowly take the arms behind you, keeping the palms upper-most and feeling a downwards stretch. Go as far as you can without straining, moving the shoulders or letting the small of your back hollow out. Repeat 5–10 times slowly.

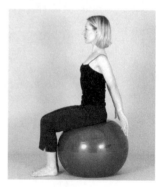

4. Sit with the arms bent at the elbows and your fingers pointing straight ahead of you. Breathe in and open the hands out to the sides, keeping the elbows tucked in to your sides. Breathe out and return to the starting position. Repeat 5–10 times, checking there is no tension in the neck or shoulders.

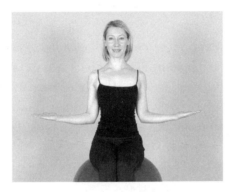

Side Stretches

This is a gentle side stretch for which you need to sit on a chair with a back that you can hold on to. Stretch as far as you can **without straining.**

1. Sit sideways on an armless chair with your feet firmly on the floor and your left hand holding the chair back. Check your back is long and straight, with your neck relaxed. Draw the navel gently to the spine and pull up the pelvic floor. Take a few slow breaths and check there is no tension anywhere in your upper body.

2. Place your right hand behind your head. Breath in and, as you breathe out, turn your head to look away from the chair back and pull up through the ribs. Now, stretch gently away from the chair back in a long curve, feeling the lower ribs stretching up, rather than sagging down.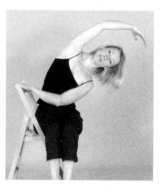

3. Breathe in to return to the starting position and repeat 5–10 times. Repeat on the other side.

Forward Bend

This exercise is adapted from yoga and contemporary dance and it is an ideal way to stretch out and release the spine. It is important that whatever you use as your support is steady enough to hold your weight without moving as you relax into the position.

**If you feel dizzy at any point during this exercise,
stop immediately.**

1. Stand facing a window ledge or heavy table or chair an arm's length away. Your feet should be firmly planted on the floor, hip-width apart. Now check your posture. Your spine should be long and straight with no tension in the neck or shoulders. Draw the navel gently to the spine and pull up the pelvic floor. Raise your arms above your head without raising your shoulders.

2. Breathe in and, as you breathe out, slowly bend forwards in one piece without letting the spine curve or arch. Feel as if you are rotating from the hips with your back long and flat. Let your fingers rest on the support and feel a long stretch through the arms, neck and back. Hold this position for up to a minute and breathe naturally.

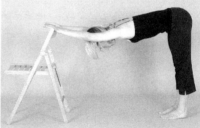

3. Now, continue the bend forwards, dropping your head down towards the floor as far as is comfortable. If this feels a strain, bend your knees slightly.

4. Breathe in and, as you breathe out, roll up slowly, feeling as if you are placing each vertebra of the spine on top of the one below until you are standing with a long, straight back. Check there is no tension in the neck, jaw or shoulders and take a few long, slow breaths. Repeat up to 5 times.

Pillow Squeeze

This is a famous Pilates exercise that combines a number of benefits. It works the pelvic floor muscles and the inner thighs, as well as helping posture awareness and relaxing the lower back. You will need a pillow or cushion for this exercise – the firmer it is, the harder you will have to work.

1. Lie on your back with your knees raised up and your feet flat on the floor. Gently hold the cushion or pillow between your knees. Place your arms by your sides, palms down. Check the shoulders and neck are relaxed and, if you are at all uncomfortable or the neck feels arched away from the floor, place a small pillow underneath your head. Breathe in, pulling up the pelvic floor muscles.

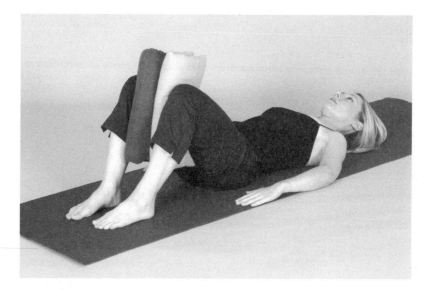

2. As you breathe out, draw the navel to the spine and squeeze the pillow with your knees, taking care not to let your back arch or tension to creep into your back, neck or shoulders. The only part of your body that should be moving is the knees.

3. Breathe in to release the cushion and repeat up to 10 times.

Relaxation Sequence

After exercising it is important for you to relax. This sequence should take between 10 and 15 minutes, depending on how you feel and how much time you have. Don't be tempted to rush it – this is a very valuable part of your routine. Even a short relaxation will make a big difference to your stress levels and overcome the feelings of tiredness that can seem overwhelming during pregnancy, as well as your ability to cope and your overall health.

The relaxation takes place in what is known in yoga as the corpse pose. Many people find it helpful to record the following instructions on tape and play it while they do the relaxation. If you do this, ensure you speak very slowly, repeating each instruction several times. During the relaxation, your body temperature will drop, so now is the time to cover yourself with a blanket or to put on an extra layer of clothing, especially socks as your feet can get cold. Make sure you are not disturbed during relaxation – turn off the phone and put a 'do not disturb' sign on the door.

Relaxation Sequence

1. Lie down on the floor with your spine long and your arms close to
   your sides, palms uppermost. It may seem more natural to face the
   palms down, but when they are facing up, the upper back and
   shoulders are lowered and not tensed and your back is more
   comfortable on the floor. Close your eyes and give yourself a few
   moments in which to become aware of the weight of your whole
   body, softening and spreading out on the floor after the exertions
   of exercising and stretching. Roll the head from side to side to
   check there is no tension in the neck.

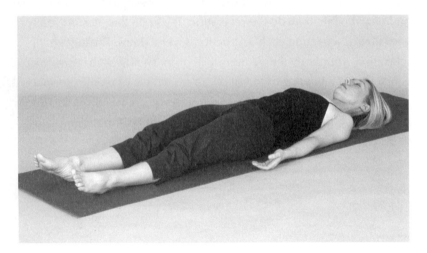

2. Starting at your toes, begin to feel the relaxation spreading through your body, moving upwards like a wave. Spend time on each tiny part, putting all your concentration into each area of your body in turn, first the toes, then the feet and ankles.

3. Feel the wave spreading up into your legs, through the shins and calves, the knees and into the thighs. Let your legs roll outwards from the hips, completely relaxed. Let the hips and buttocks go – there is often a surprising amount of tension stored here. The whole body softens and the effect now reaches the abdomen, which drops down further against the back, while the lower spine relaxes further into the floor.

4. The stomach, the waist and the ribs all expand and soften. Your breathing is now probably quite light. As the softening, relaxing wave flows through the torso and into the back, they fall deeper into the floor. The relaxation flows up into the shoulders and neck and out along the arms to the very ends of the fingers. The back of the neck is almost touching the floor, the scalp softens, almost loose against the skull, and the whole face – the jaw, the chin, the throat, the cheeks – melt away. The lips part and your tongue rests gently behind the lower teeth. The eyes sink softly back into the head and the temples and forehead smooth out.

5. The whole body is at rest. Enjoy this sensation; be aware of it. As thoughts come into your mind, watch them and see them float away like clouds in a summer sky. Any doubts or worries can float away in the same way as the physical tension has left your body. Stay in this place for 3–5 minutes. Now see the sun in your sky and feel its life-giving light and warmth. Feel the air around you and, as you take a deep breath in, feel that you are drinking in from the sun's vast source of energy, making you calmer and stronger.

6. Now begin to deepen the breath, letting the ribs expand and the lungs fill. After three breaths, begin to feel your toes and fingers coming to life. Wriggle them. Still with your eyes closed, lift your arms above your head and stretch your arms and legs away from each other. When you are ready, roll onto your side and open your eyes. Give yourself a few moments before you get up.

Alternating The Breath

After the deep relaxation of the previous exercise, a good way to restore your focus and energy is this yogic practice of alternate nostril breathing. The reason that this breathing exercise is so energizing is that, according to yoga teachings, it unblocks the flow of energy around the body. Because it improves oxygen intake, purification and circulation of the blood and lymph, oxygen flow is increased to every cell in the body. It is believed that this improves mental alertness, concentration and creativity, as well as producing a feeling of calm. It is also, quite simply, a good exercise for your lungs, strengthening the respiratory muscles.

1. Sit comfortably on the floor with your legs crossed, or in a chair with your feet flat on the floor. Whichever position you choose, it is important that your back is straight, relaxed and supported by a wall or chair back.

2. Close your eyes and breathe in. Lift your right hand up so it is level with your face and, using your thumb, close your right nostril. Exhale slowly through your left nostril and then inhale again through this nostril only.

3. Now close your left nostril with the fourth and fifth fingers. Exhale and inhale through your right nostril. Repeat the whole sequence for at least two minutes.

6

Second Trimester

During the second trimester, your body starts to change visibly – other people are now aware that you are pregnant as you begin to have a growing bump. This is often the best part of the pregnancy. Most women get over their feelings of nausea and extreme tiredness and feel very well indeed. This is the time you are most likely to glow with health (all those hormones do wonders for your skin and hair). The exercises for the second trimester build on the foundations laid in the first. Start off with the Warm-Up (page 23) and the exercises of the first trimester up to and including the Side Stretches (page 40), and then continue with these new exercises.

Warning
Some exercises in this section involve lying on your back. Some women in the later stages of pregnancy find that this is uncomfortable, or makes them feel dizzy. If lying on your back does make you uncomfortable or dizzy, do not do these exercises.

Curl-ups

This exercise builds on the pelvic floor exercises and the breathing exercises from the first trimester that helped to relax the back. Here, the back moves with the breath to increase mobility in the spine, at the same time as strengthening the pelvic and abdominal muscles.

1. Lie on your back with your knees raised, the feet slightly apart and flat on the floor. Place a rolled up towel between your knees and lengthen out the spine along the floor, with the chin tucked in a little to release and lengthen the back of the neck. Check that your shoulders and neck are relaxed, arms by your sides.

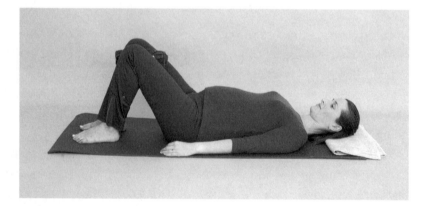

2. Take a long, slow breath in and, as you breathe out, draw the navel gently towards the spine. Squeeze the low buttock and the pelvic floor muscles and allow the back to curl up from the floor, very slowly, vertebra by vertebra. You don't need to lift off all of your back and you should always keep your shoulder blades in contact with the floor. If you lift too high, it will put a strain on your back and the aim of this exercise is to feel the mobility of the spine. Check that your shoulders and neck are relaxed.

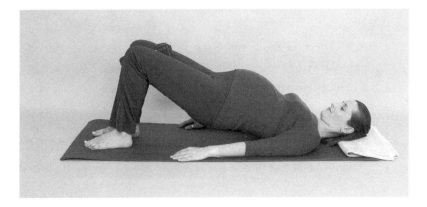

3. When you have lifted up as much as it is comfortable for your back, breathe in and, as you breathe out, lower the back down in exactly the same way, trying to feel each vertebra as you place it on the floor. Repeat 5–10 times, according to what feels comfortable.

Knee to Chest

This exercise is excellent for releasing tension in the lower back and the neck and improving the posture – but it may get more difficult as your bump gets bigger!

1. Lie on your back with your knees bent and your feet flat on the floor, the spine straight, the neck and head in the same elongated line and the chin tipped slightly downwards. Lift the knees up and feel your whole spine in contact with the floor. Place your hands just below the knees, holding them apart to fit around your bump. Draw the navel gently back towards the spine throughout the exercise.

2. Breathe in and, as you breathe out, draw your right knee towards your chest. If you keep your arms wide and rounded, this will be an expansive movement and you should feel the back opening up. Release the knee and breathe in.

3. On the next out-breath, draw the left knee to the chest in exactly the same way, checking that the spine is in contact with the floor and the neck and shoulders are relaxed.

4. As you breathe out next time, draw both knees to the chest. Repeat the whole sequence 5–10 times.

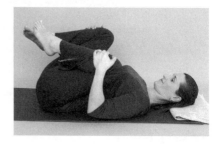

Opposite Arm and Leg Stretch

This exercise is excellent for stretching out and relaxing the body to its fullest extent.

1. Lie on your back, with your knees bent, feet flat on the floor and your arms beside you. Take a long deep breath. As you breathe out, draw the navel gently towards the spine and slide your left leg away from you onto the floor, simultaneously lifting your right arm up above your head to lie flat on the floor if possible. Try to feel the whole body – particularly the chest, shoulders, neck and back – open and relax.

2. Breathe in and, as you breathe out, return your arm and leg to the starting position. On the next out-breath, repeat with the left arm and right leg. Alternate 5–10 times.

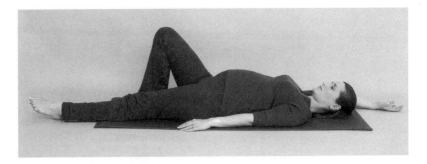

Arm Reaches

This exercise is similar to the previous one, except now it is only your arms that are alternating. This is a very useful exercise for releasing tension in the shoulders, back and neck.

1. Lying on your back, place your feet flat on the floor, slightly apart, with your knees bent. Check that your spine is straight, your chin is slightly tipped down and your neck is in alignment with your spine. Reach your arms straight up so that your fingertips are pointing at the ceiling.

2. Breathe in and, as you breathe out, take your arms in opposite directions, so that one goes above your head as close to the floor as you can manage while keeping it straight, and the other goes down to your side.

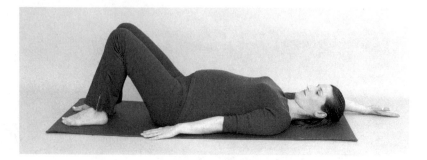

3. Stay in that position as you breathe in and then, on the out-breath, reverse the arms so the other reaches behind your head. Alternate up to 10 times.

Hip Rolls

This exercise is designed to release tension from the back and neck and it should feel relaxing. If the stretch feels too strong across your abdomen, don't roll the knees so far. And always stop if you feel any discomfort in the lower back.

1. Lie on your back with your feet together and your knees raised. Check that your neck and spine are in one long straight line, there is no hollow in the small of the back and there is no tension in the shoulders.

2. Breathe in and, as you breathe out, roll your knees gently to one side, keeping them together, but only as far as they will go without your buttocks coming off the floor.

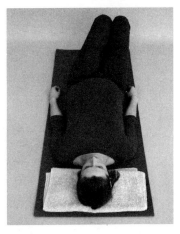

3. Breathe in to return to the centre and, as you breathe out, roll your knees to the other side. Repeat up to 10 times on each side.

Knee Drops to Side

This exercise releases the pelvic area and is a relaxing stretch when you are pregnant. Remember, however, that during pregnancy this whole area becomes much looser than normal so take care not to overstretch and don't allow the pelvis to move.

1. Lie on your back with your knees raised and your feet flat on the floor. Breathe in and, as you breathe out, gently press the navel towards the spine and drop one knee slowly to the side. Go only as far as you can without lifting the hip or moving the pelvis.

2. Breathe in and return to the starting position and, as you breathe out, drop the other knee to the side. Repeat 5 times on each side.

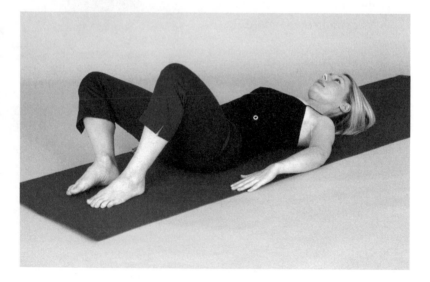

Leg Slides

This exercise mobilizes and stretches the joints of the leg. It also develops good alignment and posture.

1. Lie on the floor with your knees raised and feet together on the floor. Check your back and neck are aligned and elongated, with no tension in the shoulders and no overarching in the small of the back.

2. Breathe in and, as you breathe out, straighten one bent knee along the floor without distorting the back or the pelvis. Make it a long, slow stretch throughout the leg and foot, pointing the toe. Breathe in and return to the starting position.

3. Repeat with the other leg on the next out-breath and alternate 5 times on each side.

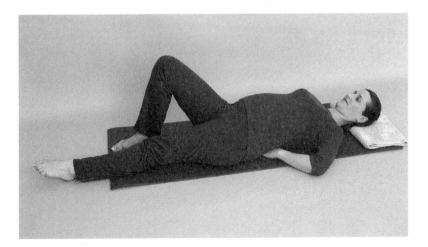

Hamstring Stretch OEDEMA

This is a gentle stretch for the hamstrings (the muscles in the backs of the thighs) and helps to relieve the feeling of heavy legs during pregnancy. Don't overdo it, though, just take the leg as far as you need in order to feel the stretch without any straining in the lower back.

1. Lie on your back with an elongated spine, raised knees and feet flat on the floor. Check that your shoulders are relaxed and you are not overarching in the back. Bring your left knee up towards your chest and wrap a long scarf or belt around the foot.

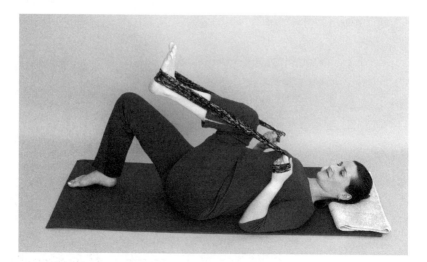

2. Take a long breath in and, as you breathe out, gently draw the navel towards the spine and straighten the leg up towards the ceiling. The knee should be facing you and the neck and shoulders should remain relaxed. Don't pull hard on your leg, it will just distort your pelvis and back. You should be feeling a stretch not pain. Hold the stretch for a count of 10–20, breathing normally and flexing the foot if you find it too easy (this increases the stretch).

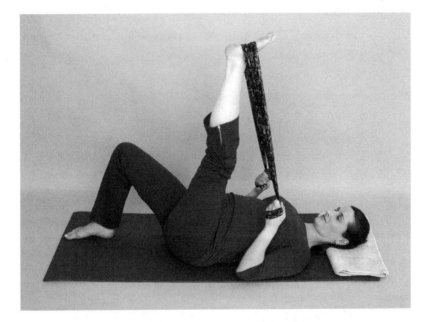

3. Bend the leg and relax for a moment, then repeat on the other side.

Leg Stretches

This is one of the most famous original Pilates exercises, adapted for pregnancy. Post-pregnancy, there is another version that is a little more demanding to get your abdominal muscles back in shape (*see page* 117).

1. Lie on your back with your feet together flat on the floor and your knees raised. Now take your feet off the floor, keeping the knees apart to make a V-shape towards your toes. Check that your back is flat on the floor and your neck and shoulders are relaxed.

2. Breathe in and bring one knee up towards your chest. Then, as you breathe out, draw the navel to the spine, making sure the whole spine is on the floor and stretch up the second leg, pointing the toe. Check that the spine is still elongated along the floor and there is no tension in the neck or shoulders.

3. Take another long full breath and, as you breathe out, change the legs so the second leg is drawn in towards the chest and the first is stretched up. Always keep the whole back on the floor. If you feel any discomfort stop immediately. Alternate 5–10 times on each side.

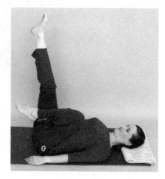

Leg Lifts OEDEMA ✓

Gently exercising the legs during pregnancy helps to reduce swelling and keeps the muscles strong. It is best to practise this exercise with your back against a wall to ensure your spine stays in complete alignment.

1. Lie on your side, preferably against a wall with a big cushion beneath your upper leg, and smaller ones (or rolled up towels) to support your waist. Make sure that your back is flat against the wall. Stretch out your lower arm parallel to your spine, placing a cushion between it and your head. Bend your lower leg and flex the foot of your upper leg on the cushions.

2. Place your upper hand on your upper hip and take a long breath in. As you breathe out, draw the navel gently to the spine and feel the shoulder blades draw down and the neck lengthen. Lengthen out along your upper side and bring your top leg up in a low lift, making sure the whole leg – foot, knee and hip – is facing forwards. The feeling to aim at is a long stretch rather than an actual lift.

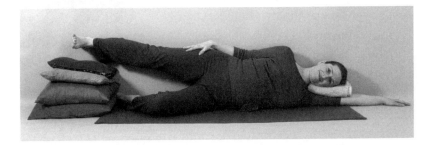

3. Do 5-10 lifts on this side and then repeat on the other.

The Cossack

The best way to do this exercise is in front of a mirror so that you can check your position. It is a very helpful exercise for learning how your spine works and for improving your posture generally. Remember to keep the spine lengthened and aligned throughout, with the navel drawn gently towards the backbone.

1. Sit squarely on a ball or chair in front of a mirror with your arms folded a few inches in front of the chest. Rest your hands against your arms – don't grip as this will create tension in the shoulders. Breathe in and feel the whole spine drawn gently up through the top of the head, as if you were a puppet on a string.

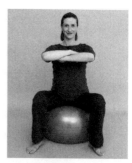

2. As you breathe out, turn – as if your spine were a pivot – feeling the turn begin at the bottom of the spine, up through the back to the shoulders and, finally, the head. Don't let the hips move – they should face straight to the front throughout.

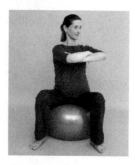

3. Breathe in and return to the starting position and, as you breathe out, turn to the other side. Alternate, 5 times on each side.

Squatting Against a Wall

This exercise originates from a yoga exercise and is perfect for the later stages of pregnancy as it relaxes and increases the mobility of the pelvic and hip joints. Many women find this a very comfortable position, as well as being a favoured position for giving birth. **Do not do this exercise, however, if your baby is in the breech position.**

1. Put a large cushion on the floor next to a wall. Stand against the wall so that your lower back is touching it and your feet are a hip-width apart.

2. Breathe in and, as you breathe out, begin to bend your knees and gradually slide your lower back down the wall. Keep your heels flat on the floor and, if you find you cannot get down to the cushion, add another, or use a low stool. When your bottom reaches the cushion, lean your arms on to your knees and rest in this position.

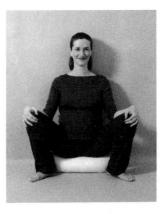

3. Stay in this position for a minute or two and try to feel the weight drop down through the feet and buttocks and let your back relax. When you are ready, take a deep breath in and on the out-breath, slide slowly back up the wall.

The Cat

Being on all fours is a comfortable position in pregnancy and becomes even more so as the months pass. Simply holding the first 'table top' position, below, is an excellent exercise as you start to get bigger and takes the weight of the baby off your back for a while. This exercise stretches and releases the back and the best way of doing it is as slowly and smoothly as possible, allowing one position to blend into the next. If you have any back problems, however, only do the first two positions.

1. If possible, do this exercise next to a mirror so you can check that your back is completely flat. Position yourself on your hands and knees, with your knees a hip-width apart, and check that your shoulders, hips and knees are all in alignment. Try to make your back perfectly flat with no tension in the neck and your head relaxed and in line with the spine.

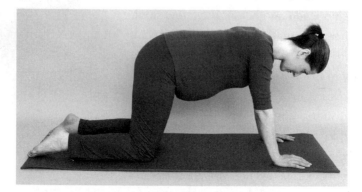

2. Breathe in and, as you breathe out, gently draw the navel back towards the spine so that your back arches upwards and your head drops down between your arms, keeping them straight as you do so. Breathe in and return to the position above.

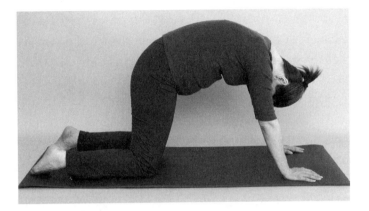

3. Breathe out and arch your back the other way so that it hollows out with your head and your bottom the highest points of your body. Breathe in and return to position 1. Repeat 5–10 times.

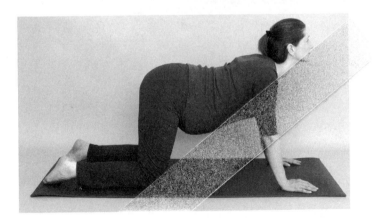

Cushion Squeeze

This is essentially a relaxation exercise though it also tones up the inner thighs. The harder the cushion, the better it works.

1. Lie on your back with an elongated spine, the navel drawn gently towards the spine, the knees raised and the feet, slightly apart, flat on the floor. Place a cushion between the knees and thighs.

2. Breathe in and, as you breathe out, pull in the muscles of the buttocks and thighs and squeeze the cushion to the count of 10. Repeat 5–10 times.

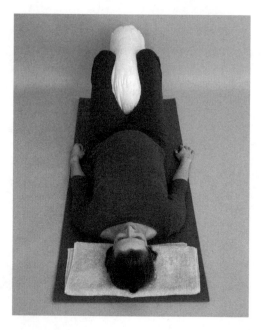

Relaxation Sequence

Finish your exercise session with the Relaxation Sequence given on page 45.

7

Third Trimester

By the end of the third trimester you are carrying around 20 lbs (or 9 kg) of extra weight. Not surprisingly, particularly towards the end of the pregnancy, many women start to feel very tired, or sometimes breathless, and can't wait for it to end! There are other specific problems that you may find during this final stage of pregnancy. One is oedema, where the hands, feet and ankles swell up with excess fluid. You can reduce oedema with exercises in this section designed to bring mobility to specific areas and so reduce water retention in them. Your digestive system does not have much room to function and you may find it slows down, resulting in constipation or heartburn. Gentle exercise and drinking plenty of water will help in both cases. Finally, some, though not all women finding lying on their back uncomfortable during the last six weeks or so of pregnancy. If so, avoid any exercises that use this position. Start your session with the Warm-Up exercises (*see page* 23), as much as you find comfortable of the routine for the second trimester up to the Cat (page 66) and add the following exercises, as you feel able.

Warning

Some exercises in this section involve lying on your back. Some women in the later stages of pregnancy find that this is uncomfortable, or makes them feel dizzy. If lying on your back does make you uncomfortable or dizzy, do not do these exercises.

Foot Arching OEDEMA

During the last three months of pregnancy, the risk of oedema increases, causing swelling especially in the feet and ankles. Keeping your feet raised whenever possible is a good idea. Support them on a cushion if you are lying down on a bed or sofa, and try this exercise and the wall support exercises, too.

1. Sit fairly near the edge of a chair, with your feet slightly apart and flat on the floor and your knees bent at right angles. Check that your back is straight, your head held high as an extension of the spine, and that your shoulders and neck are relaxed. Place your hands on your thighs.

2. Without moving your heels, slowly draw back your toes so that your insteps lift up and the arches increase.

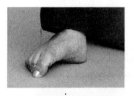

3. Slide the toes back to the starting position and, keeping the soles of the feet in contact with the floor, stretch the toes upwards as far as they will go. Repeat the sequence 10 times.

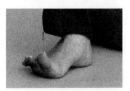

4. Wiggle your toes in a wave motion – the Mexican wave!

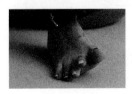

Foot Massage

Massage not only feels wonderful, but it also helps to soothe the feet in pregnancy when they have to carry so much more weight than usual. If you have a friend or partner who will massage your feet it is a real treat, but you can easily do it yourself – either after you have been exercising or just before you go to bed, when it often improves your sleep.

1. Sitting on a chair so that you can bend your knees at right angles, place one calf on the other thigh so that the foot is in easy reach. Start by gently stroking the whole of your foot and squeezing out any obvious areas of tension.
2. Rotate your ankle 5 times clockwise, then 5 times anticlockwise. Using both thumbs, apply a firm pressure all over the sole of the foot, then at the top of the foot and the ankles.

3. Gently pull each toe to give it a comfortable stretch. Repeat with the other foot.

Ankle Exercise

This is another good exercise for soothing tired, swollen feet.

1. Sit with your back against the wall and your feet raised, your lower legs supported on a cushion. Making sure that your feet are in line with your legs (no pigeon toes!), stretch your feet as far as you can without your legs coming off the cushion. Point and stretch your toes and hold for a count of 5.

2. Bring your feet back to the starting position but continue the movement so that the feet flex – the toes pointing up to the ceiling and the heels pushing away. Hold for a count of 5. Repeat both steps 5 times.

3. Now circle the ankles 5 times clockwise, then 5 times anticlockwise.

Hand and Wrist Exercise

Oedema can affect the hands and wrists, too, so that fingers swell up and rings feel tight. This exercise helps reduce swelling and tension.

1. Sit comfortably on a chair or on the floor, with your back supported and no tension in your neck or shoulders. Bring your hands together in a prayer position and then open them up so that only the fingertips are touching. Push the fingertips together firmly without any other parts of the hands touching. Hold for a count of 10.

2. Holding your hands loosely in front of you, shake them 10 times.

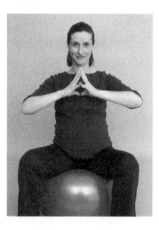

3. Make a loose fist and fling open then close your hands 10 times, really pointing your fingers.

4. Rotate your wrists 5 times clockwise, then 5 times anticlockwise.

Arm Raises

This exercise helps to improve posture, as well as loosening tense necks and shoulders. You need a long scarf for this one.

1. Stand with your feet hip-width apart, with a long straight back and neck. Draw the navel gently towards the spine to eliminate any overarching and keep that feeling there throughout the exercise.

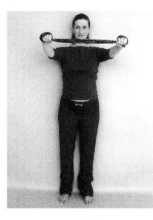

2. Hold the scarf lightly taut in front of you with your hands about a metre apart. Breathe in and, as you breathe out, raise the scarf until it is above your head, without allowing a hollow to appear in your lower back. Don't lift your shoulders as you raise your arms. Instead feel the movement coming from your shoulder blades. Keep the neck and shoulders soft and relaxed throughout.

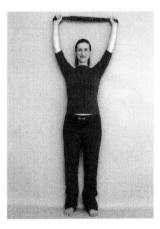

3. At the top, breathe in then, as you breathe out, lower the scarf again. Repeat 5 times.

Legs Against The Wall

This is another position in which both to stretch and relax during late pregnancy. It also helps reduce swelling in the ankles and feet. Do not go on to the second position unless you are quite comfortable in the first, and you feel no strain in the lower back.

1. With a cushion for your head, position yourself so that your bottom is touching the wall. It is probably easiest to approach the wall by rolling sideways into position and bending your knees down towards your body. Check that your back is long and relaxed, and then walk your legs up the wall as far as is comfortable. If they will stretch effortlessly, straighten the legs and flex the feet, otherwise keep the toes pointed and the knees as bent as you need. Do not arch the lower back. Hold this position for 5 minutes – longer if you have time.

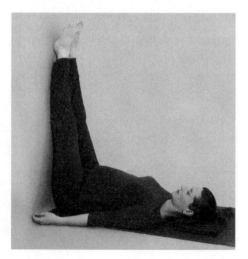

2. If you find the first position easy, you can add to it by creating a stretch for the inner thighs. Gradually let your legs fall outwards to the sides until you feel a stretch, but not a strain. If your lower back comes off the floor, bring the legs closer together until it is flat again. Relax in this position for 5 minutes.

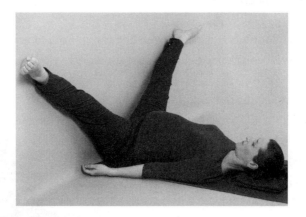

3. Bend the knees and roll sideways onto the floor to come out of either position.

Spinal Twist

This is both a relaxing exercise for the back and a stretch for the hamstring and calf muscles. Don't overdo it, though - go just as far as it remains a stretch **without becoming a strain.**

1. Sit on the floor with your legs stretched out in front of you. Sit up straight with a long back and relaxed shoulders.

2. Bend your left leg and cross your foot over your right leg. Keep it by the side of your right knee, keeping your left knee bent up in front of you.

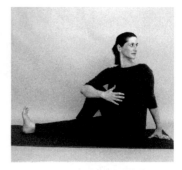

3. Hold onto your left knee with your right arm.

4. Place the palm of your left hand on the floor behind you.

5. Turn your head to look over your left shoulder.

6. Slowly turn back to the centre and repeat the exercise on the other leg.

Sitting with Legs Wide Apart

This is very similar to the Legs Against The Wall exercise on page 78 and, strictly speaking, it is not so much an exercise but more of a sitting position that is particularly comfortable in late pregnancy. It does, however, stretch the inner thighs and hamstrings, increase mobility in the hip joints and release tension in the back and shoulders. It is also a good position to use for breathing exercises – or just watching television!

1. Sit with your lower back supported by a wall, legs straight out in front. Feel your spine very long and straight, with your head well supported.

2. Without distorting your back, open your legs wide enough apart to feel a stretch but not so far as to feel a strain. Sit, breathe deeply and relax into the position. If you want to increase the stretch, you can either take the legs farther apart, or flex the feet.

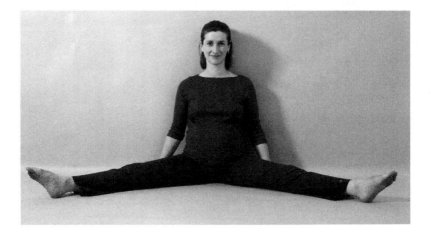

Leg Raises with Pillow Support

This exercise keeps the legs toned, while giving a certain amount of comfort and support.

1. Sit on the floor with your back supported by the wall and your legs straight out in front of you. Place a double pillow under your right knee so that it supports the leg and place the left foot on the floor with the knee bent.

2. Slowly straighten the right leg, point the toe, flex the heel and lower the leg to the cushion. Repeat this 10 times and then change legs.

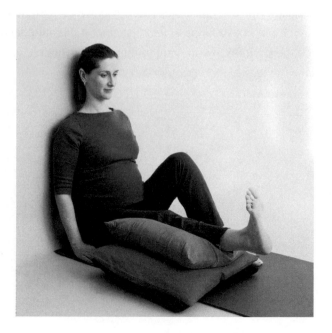

Child's Pose with Pillow Support

This is a very good relaxation position in late pregnancy as it relieves the pressure on the lower back and opens up the pelvic area. Use a lot of cushions for comfort.

1. Sit on top of a cushion or bolster with your knees as open as possible and your feet close to your buttocks. Have a large cushion (or heap of cushions) in front of you. Make sure your spine is straight and lengthened and there is no tension in the neck or shoulders. Close your eyes and take 5 deep, slow breaths and feel your whole body relax.

2. Place your hands on the floor and walk your body to the cushions in front of you, placing your arms and head on top and relaxing into the pose. Keep your back long and place your head to one side if that is more comfortable. Try to feel all of your muscles and joints soften and relax and breathe slowly and comfortably for a few minutes. Return to the starting position slowly and sit with your eyes closed, breathing deeply.

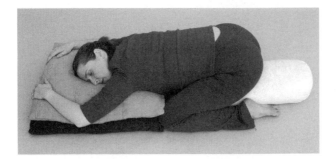

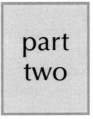

part
two

Exercising After the Birth

Exercising After the Birth

Immediately after the birth you are likely to be feeling a combination of joy and excitement, tempered by extreme tiredness. This tiredness is likely to increase over the next few days and weeks with sleepless nights and the constant demands of a new baby. At first, then, exercise is going to be the last thing on your mind, but there is one sequence of exercises you should start to do as soon as possible – pelvic floor exercises (*see pages* 28). You can do these in bed if you wish, but do try to start within days of the birth if you can.

The exercises in this part of the book are divided into three sections: the first three months, three to six months, and six months and onwards. These are only to be used as a very approximate guide. Don't do anything (except for pelvic floor exercises) until you have been given the all-clear after your six-week check-up. If you have had a Caesarean section, you will need to wait quite a bit longer, certainly to do any exercises that use the abdominal muscles. If you have had a Caesarean, don't start until your doctor tells you that you're ready.

When you start working through the exercises, don't feel you must rush on to the next section because you have reached the three-month or six-month point. As with all Pilates exercises, you should only progress on to the next stage when you are completely confident with your current exercises. If, when you do try a new exercise, you feel it is a strain, stop. You are not ready and you could do more harm than good by pushing yourself too hard at this stage. Keep practising at your previous level until you are stronger.

If you are starting Pilates for the first time after you have had your baby, go back and make sure you can do all the exercises in the pregnancy section first. These early stages were vital for laying the foundations of your technique, so you need to do these to ensure you are doing the later, more complex, exercises correctly.

8

First Three Months After the Birth

As soon as you can after the birth, start the pelvic floor exercises (page 28) and do them as often as you remember. If breast-feeding is giving you tension in the shoulders or neck, do the Head Rolls and Tilts (page 33) and Shoulder Lifts and Circles (page 35). When you have had the go-ahead from your doctor to start exercising again, repeat the Warm-up and the exercises for the first trimester then, as you feel able, add the following new exercises.

Pointing and Flexing The Feet

There are two ways of doing this particular exercise. Both will tone your legs and buttocks as well as your abdominal muscles and reduce any fluid retention in the ankles. You can sit on the floor or, alternatively you can use a ball, making your abdominal muscles work even harder to keep your balance. Start with the first version.

1. Sit on the floor with your legs stretched out in front of you. Feel a stretch through the whole length of the leg. Check that your back is straight, the navel pulled in gently towards the spine and that you are sitting up on your 'sitting bones', engaging the gluteal muscles in your buttocks. Your shoulders should be dropped with the arms out-stretched in front of you at shoulder height.

2. Maintaining exactly the same position, flex the feet so that the toes point up to the ceiling. The heels may come off the floor if you are pushing hard enough. Keep your knees facing the ceiling. Point and flex 10–20 times.

Variation

Stand, holding onto a chair back, with the same straight back as before. Draw the navel gently to the spine and raise one foot from the floor. Point and flex 10–20 times, then repeat with the other foot.

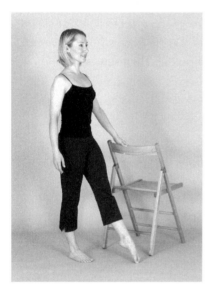 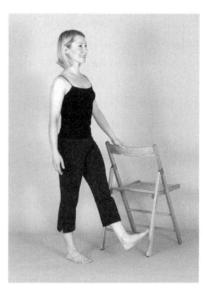

Arm Toner 1

This exercise, and the one that follows, looks deceptively easy. In fact, when you do it properly, it is quite hard work and very effective at toning the upper arms and getting rid of any excess fluid retention. It is important that the effort takes place in the arms and hands. Don't let tension creep into the neck and shoulders. They should stay relaxed, while the arms are moved from the back, keeping the shoulders themselves still.

1. Sit with your legs loosely crossed in front of you – put a small cushion under your bottom if you don't feel comfortable in this position on the floor. Draw the navel to the spine, lift up out of the waist and hips – feel there is space between your ribs – and stretch the arms out, making a loose fist, a few inches off the floor.

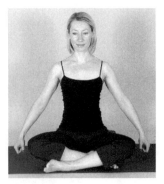

2. Fling out your fingers as far as they will go, raising your arms slightly as you do so. Then make another fist as you raise the arms again. Repeat, alternating flings and fists, taking up to ten movements to get to the top, with your arms stretching up above your head. Make sure your shoulders do not lift as your arms get higher.

3. Repeat the same pattern to bring the arms down and, if you find the exercise quite easy, repeat up to five times.

Arm Toner 2

This is another excellent way of toning the arms. Again, it is vital to keep the shoulders dropped and the neck relaxed. If you feel tension creeping in, stop, do some shoulder circles and start again.

1. Sit with your legs loosely crossed, using a cushion to sit on if necessary. Draw the navel towards your spine, which should be long and straight, with relaxed shoulders and neck. Without lifting the shoulders stretch your arms out to the sides at shoulder height.

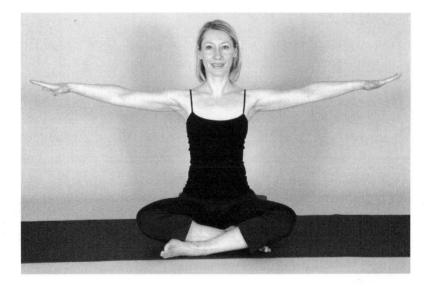

2. Flex the hands back as hard as you can so that the fingers are straight, pointing up towards the ceiling. You will feel a stretch all the way along the underside of the arms.

3. Reverse the hands so they drop down, curling the fingers back towards your body as far as they will go. You should feel a strong stretch along the backs of the hands, wrists and forearms. Flex and curl 10–20 times. If you feel any tension, do some shoulder circles to release the muscles.

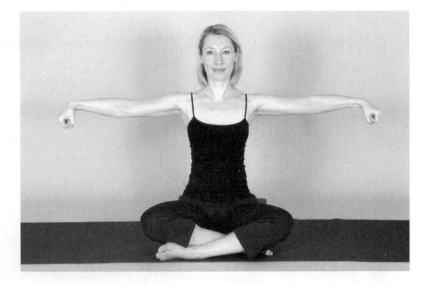

'Walking' On Your Bottom

This is another bottom and leg-toning exercise. For maximum effect, 'step' as far as you can every time.

1. Sit on the floor with a long straight back, navel drawn to the spine and shoulders and neck relaxed. Sit up on your sitting bones, gluteal muscles engaged, and with your legs in a long stretch in front of you, right through to your toes. Stretch your arms out in front of you at shoulder height or 'march' them in time with your legs.

2. Moving from the hip and keeping the back straight, 'walk' the right leg forwards so that the right foot is in front of the left. Now 'walk' the left leg in front of the right. Repeat forwards for ten steps, then backwards for another ten.

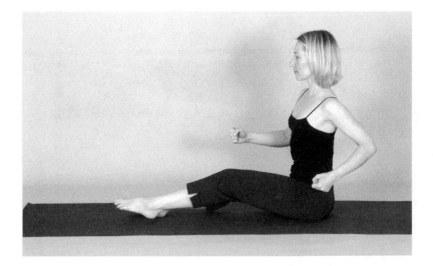

The Scoop

The scoop is based on the breathing exercise that you did during pregnancy (*see page* 30). Now, though, it turns into a pelvic tilt to work the abdominal muscles. It is also a good way of incorporating your pelvic floor exercises into your routine – they work perfectly with this exercise.

1. Lie on your back on the floor with your knees raised to the ceiling and your feet flat on the floor, a hip-width apart. Check that your back is long and straight and there is no tension in the shoulders, neck or face. Place your arms a little apart from your sides, with the palms face down.

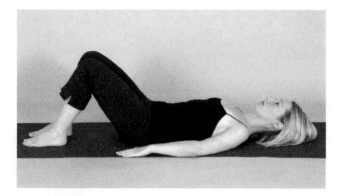

2. Breathe in and, as you breathe out, draw the navel to the spine, squeeze the pelvic floor and the low buttock muscles and feel the abdomen hollow out into a shallow scoop. This movement takes place only in the lower body – your upper body should remain still and without any tension.

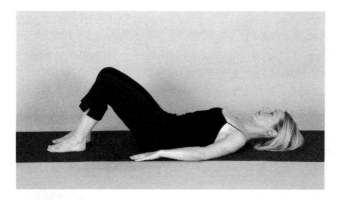

3. Repeat up to 10 times, each time trying to extend the movement. If your abdominal muscles are strong enough, you can curl up the lower buttocks very slightly from the floor. Keep the lower back on the floor at all times, though, and if you feel any strain, don't try to take the buttocks off the floor either.

Side Rolls

This exercise gently works the spine and the oblique abdominal muscles. If you find it too hard at first with a tennis ball try it without, but keep the knees together and level.

1. Lie on your back with your knees raised and your spine long and straight on the floor. Place your arms at a 45° angle to your body, palms facing upwards, with no tension in the shoulders or neck. Place a tennis ball between your knees with your feet the same distance apart.

2. Breathe in and, as you breathe out, start to roll your knees slowly in one direction, your head in the other. Your feet will turn on to their sides but they should not come off the floor. Keep both shoulders on the floor throughout. Use your abdominal muscles to control the movement and don't let your back arch.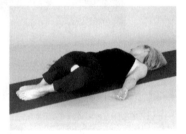

3. When you have turned as far as you can without straining, breathe in. As you breathe out, come back to the centre, again using the abdominal muscles to roll the ribs, then the back, then the buttocks on to the floor. Check that your shoulders have not lifted or tensed. Now repeat in the other direction slowly. Repeat up to 10 times.

Buttock Squeeze

This exercise tones the lower abdominal and buttock muscles. Strengthening these muscles protects the back, which has been under a particular strain during pregnancy. It is important not to arch in the lower back or let any tension creep in to the back, neck or shoulders. The top part of the body should be completely relaxed throughout.

1. Lie face down on the floor with a pillow underneath your abdomen and a smaller one between your thighs. Rest your forehead on your hands, turning your head to one side if that is more comfortable. Your shoulders and neck should be relaxed.

2. Breathe in and, as you breathe out, draw your navel off the cushion, pressing it back towards the spine and, at the same time, squeeze the cushions between the thighs using the muscles at the base of the buttocks and the inner thighs. Hold for a count of 5–10 and release. Check that there is no tension in your upper body and repeat up to 5 times.

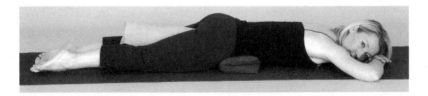

Variation

When you can do this with ease, remove the cushion from under the abdomen and do the same exercise, keeping the abdominal muscles lifted throughout.

Heel Lifts

This exercise follows on naturally from the last one as you are lying in exactly the same position, with your abdominal muscles supported by a cushion. You do not, though, have a cushion between the thighs. The more slowly you do this exercise, the more effective it will be.

1. Lie face down, as in the previous exercise. Breathe in and, as you breathe out, draw the navel to the spine and squeeze the pelvic floor muscles and the same buttock muscles that you used in the Buttock Squeeze (above). Check there is no tension in the upper body and hold this position for the rest of the exercise.

2. Breathe in and, as you breathe out, bend the right leg with a flexed foot as far as you can towards the right buttock. Move slowly and feel the stretch in the hamstring while you hold on firmly to the abdominal and buttock muscles.

3. Breathe in, lower the foot, and repeat – with the correct breathing – 10 times on each side, always checking that you are still holding on to the abdominal and buttock muscles.

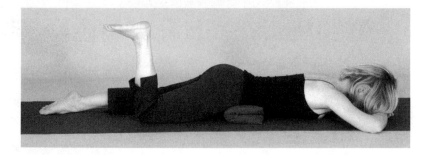

Alternate Arm and Leg Stretches

This exercise continues to work on the central girdle of strength, as well as toning and stretching the arms and legs. The pillow is there to remind you to keep lifting the abdominal muscles away from the floor – when you get stronger, you should be able to take away the cushion and leave a gap between you and the floor.

1. Lie face down with a cushion under the abdominal muscles, as in the previous exercise. Stretch your arms above your head, palms facing the floor, and place your feet a hip-width apart, the knees facing the floor. Check that your neck and shoulders are relaxed. Breathe in and, as you breathe out, draw the navel to the spine and hold this position throughout the exercise.

2. Breathe in and, as you breathe out, squeeze the pelvic floor muscles and stretch out the right arm and the left leg as far as you can, keeping them low to the floor. When you have stretched as much as possible, breathe in and lower to the floor.

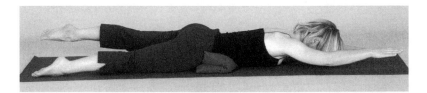

3. Breathe in and, as you breathe out, stretch the left arm and the right leg as far as you can. Check that there is no tension in the neck, shoulders or jaw and that the navel is still strong and drawn in to the spine. Then repeat the whole sequence up to 5 times.

Bottom Toner

This exercise continues to work the girdle of strength, while toning the gluteal muscles in the buttocks.

1. Lie face down on the floor with the cushion under your abdominal muscles, as before. Fold your arms in front of you and place your forehead on top of them. Turn your face to one side if that is more comfortable. Breathe in and, as you breathe out, draw the navel to the spine, trying to lift it above the cushion. Hold this position for the rest of the exercise.

2. Stretch out your right leg, pointing the toes, so that it comes off the ground. Now lift the leg further so that you squeeze the pelvic floor muscles and the buttock, but without hollowing the lower back, or letting any tension creep in to the upper body.

3. Lift 10 times on each side, and then repeat the whole sequence with a flexed foot, the toes pointing straight down to the floor.

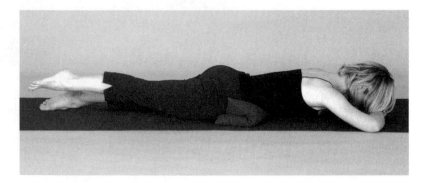

Standing Side Stretch

This simple stretch works several different areas. It helps improve posture, uses the girdle of strength and stretches out the whole of the upper body. You need a firm support to hold on to – a heavy table or chair, for instance.

1. Stand side-on to your support with your hand resting gently on it. Start by standing close to the support for a gentle stretch; then, as you become stronger and more supple, move further away for a greater stretch. Place your feet hip-width apart, check there is no tension anywhere in the body. Take a few deep breaths and try to feel yourself growing taller, by lengthening the spine so you can feel space between the ribs.

2. Breathe in and, as you breathe out, draw the navel to the spine and lift the outer arm in a wide circle up and over your head bending your body away from the support. Keep facing forwards the whole time, and don't let your hips or shoulders turn to face the support. You should feel a stretch all the way through your side.

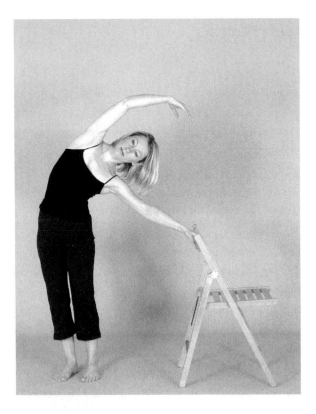

3. Breathe in to return to the starting position. Check there is no tension in the upper body and that the shoulders are dropped, and repeat up to 10 times on each side.

Twist with a Swing

Before you begin these twists, do the Cossack exercise (*see page* 64) a few times first, to check your posture and the rotation of the spine.

1. Stand very tall with the spine elongated and the upper body relaxed. Breathe in and, as you breathe out, draw the navel to the spine. With your arms at your sides rotate around the spine, turning from the waist and letting your arms swing as they follow the movement. Don't move your arms on purpose, though. Swing a few times on each side, alternating between them.

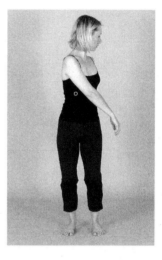

2. Make the swing looser still by bending your knees each time you come back to the centre. Keep the knees and hips facing front all the time – only your upper body moves. Repeat 10 times on each side, feeling the neck, shoulders and arms loose and free.

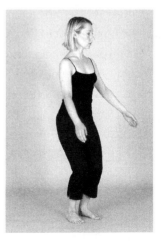

Turn-out Exercise

This looks like an exercise for the feet and ankles, but it's actually much more than that as it rotates the whole leg within the hip joint and firms up the thighs and buttocks.

1. Stand with your feet together, holding on to a firm support. Stand very tall with the spine elongated and the upper body relaxed. Breathe in and, as you breathe out, draw the navel to the spine, pull up the pelvic floor muscles and tuck in the buttocks and very slowly turn the feet out keeping the knees in line with the feet. Start the movement from the hips and feel the whole leg rotate, not just the feet or ankles.

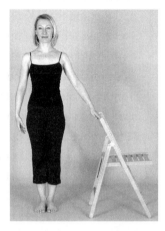

2. Reverse the movement bringing your feet back to parallel. Keep a firm hold on your abdominal muscles throughout this exercise or you will start to arch the lower back. Repeat 10 times.

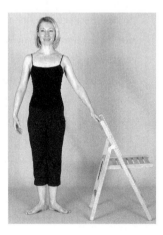

Foot Exercise

To keep your balance in this exercise, you need to work your girdle of strength. If you find it difficult not to wobble, use a support to hold on to, at least at first. As your core strength and balance improve, though, you won't need one.

1. Stand tall, with one hand lightly on a support if necessary. Check there is no tension in the upper body. Breathe in and, as you breathe out, draw the navel gently to the spine and tuck the buttocks in slightly to prevent any arching in the back. Hold this position throughout the exercise.

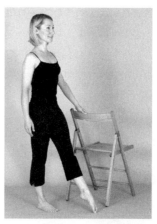

2. Take your right foot forward with a pointed toe. Now lift and flex the heel, put the toe back on to the floor and draw it back to the other leg. Repeat 5–10 times and then repeat on the left.

Variation

When you can do this with ease, make a circle with a pointed toe, 4 times clockwise, then 4 times anticlockwise on each side.

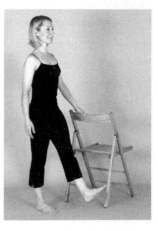

Cushion Squeeze

Follow the foot exercise with the Cushion Squeeze exercise, as on page 68.

Relaxation Sequence

Finish your exercise session with the Relaxation Sequence given on page 45.

9

Three to Six Months After the Birth

You are now probably absorbed by the new rhythm of your life as you take care of your baby. You may still be having broken sleep at night and you do still need to rest when you feel the need. You are also probably anxious to get back into shape and more aware of the imperfections of your post-baby body. The main thing now is not to rush. You will get your figure back but your ligaments are still soft and it is easy to strain them at this stage, particularly as you are probably doing a lot more lifting and carrying of your baby and countless other things – cots, prams, etc. Continue with the exercises from the previous section up to the Cushion Squeeze and, as you feel stronger, introduce the following new ones.

Pliés

Pliés originate, of course, in ballet. They may look like simple knee bends but, performed properly, they are much more than that. They are excellent at toning the legs but it is important to keep the back straight, the navel drawn to the spine and the shoulders relaxed throughout.

1. Stand in a good posture, with a long, straight back, the neck long, the shoulders relaxed and dropped down into the back. Use the back of a chair as support if you need to. Breathe in and, as you breathe out, draw the navel to the spine, feeling the back lengthen out even more.

2. On the next out-breath, turn the feet out into a V-shape, feeling the muscles in the thighs turning out from the tops of the legs. You should feel as if your inner thigh is trying to face the front! This will also make you engage the buttock muscles. Don't try to take the toes too far. Your knees should be directly over your feet. Check that you are not arching in the spine.

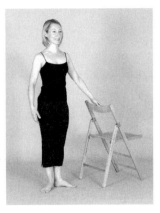

3. Breathe in and, as you breathe out, bend the knees without letting the heels lift off from the floor, 'wrapping around' the thigh muscles even more and lengthening the spine as you go down. Feel as if the spine is lengthening so much that you are trying to maintain the same height even though your knees are bent. If your knees are rolling in and are not directly above the feet, bring the toes closer together.

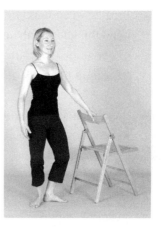

4. Breathe in and come up and, as you straighten the legs, keep on going so that you rise up onto your toes. Repeat slowly up to 10 times.

5. Take the feet about 18 inches apart, maintaining the same posture. Again, the knees should be in line with the feet. The muscles work in exactly the same way as before, with the thigh muscles wrapping around, the inner thighs trying to face forwards. It can be hard to keep the back straight in this position so check sideways in a mirror to make sure that you are not arching when you move.

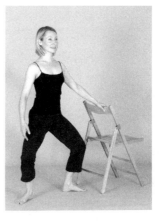

6. Breathe in and, as you breathe out, draw the navel to the spine and bend the knees only as far as they will go without taking the heels off the floor. Check that the knees are not rolling in and there is no tension in the neck or shoulders.

7. Breathe in and straighten the legs, continuing the stretch into a rise. Repeat slowly up to 10 times.

Quad Stretch

The quadriceps are the muscles at the front of your thighs (the hamstrings are the ones at the back). After working them in the previous exercise, you need to stretch them out.

Stand very tall with your shoulders dropped, your navel drawn gently to the spine and the back long and straight. If you feel you might lose your balance, hold on to a heavy chair or table. Bend the right knee and take the foot behind you, holding the ankle with one or both hands. Try to align the two knees, but don't let the back arch. Hold the stretch for up to a minute, and then change legs.

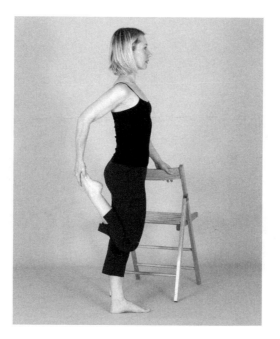

Hamstring Stretch

Sit on the floor with a long, straight back and relaxed shoulders, your legs stretched out in front of you. Take your left foot and place it against your right thigh, letting the left leg relax. Breathe in and, as you breathe out, reach forwards along your right leg, keeping your back long and straight and the shoulders dropped down into your back. Try not to strain or round the back as this will tense up the shoulders. Take a series of long, deep breaths, each time trying to reach further down the leg. If you find this very difficult, use a long scarf wound around your foot to help ease you down. Repeat on the other side.

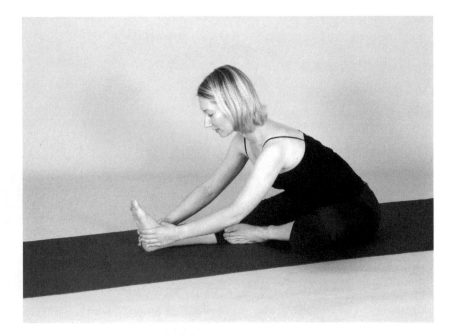

Gluteal Stretch

When you have worked the legs, it is a good idea to stretch out these muscles.

Lie on your back with your knees bent and your feet flat on the floor. Place your left ankle over the right knee then lift the right leg so that the left leg presses towards you. You will feel a stretch up the back of the left thigh and into the buttocks. Press only as far as a stretch – not a strain. Hold for a count of 20 and lower. Repeat on the other leg.

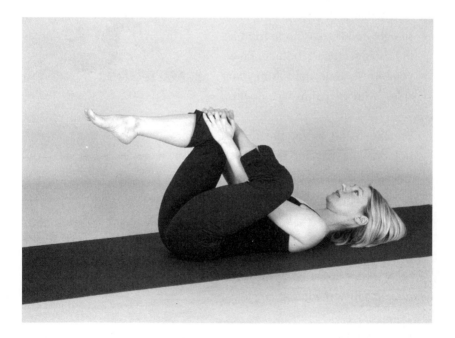

Pelvic Tilts

This exercise builds on the Scoop (*see page* 96) but you now have your feet raised up on a chair. Always use the Scoop as a warm-up for this exercise and start with just one or two repetitions, building up gradually. It is important that you don't try to come up too far. If your lower back begins to arch or the abdominal or thigh muscles quiver, come back down to the floor. Keep the movement slow and controlled throughout.

1. Lie on your back on the floor with your feet on a stable chair. Check that your back is long and straight and there is no tension in the shoulders, neck or face. Place your arms a little apart from your sides, with the palms face down.

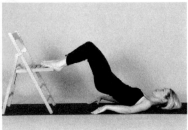

2. Breathe in and, as you breathe out, draw the navel to the spine, squeeze the pelvic floor and the low buttock muscles and feel the abdomen hollow out into a shallow scoop. This movement takes place only in the lower body – your upper body should remain still and without any tension.

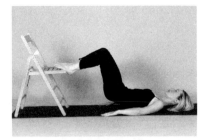

3. Keeping the scooped-out shape, curl up the lower buttocks from the floor. Repeat up to 10 times.

Single Leg Stretches

During pregnancy, you were introduced to a less demanding version of this exercise. Post-pregnancy, this version gets your abdominal muscles back in shape.

1. Lie on your back with your feet flat on the floor and your knees raised. Now draw your knees to your chest, keeping them apart to make a V-shape towards your toes. Check that your back is flat on the floor and your neck and shoulders are relaxed.

2. Breathe in and bring one knee up towards your chest. Then, as you breathe out, draw the navel to the spine, making sure the whole spine is on the floor, pull up the pelvic floor muscles and stretch out the second leg in front of you with a pointed toe. Check that the 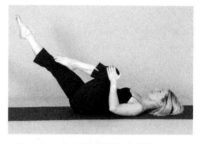 spine is still elongated along the floor and there is no tension in the neck or shoulders. The closer the leg is to the floor, the more effort the abdominal muscles will have to make. However, if the lower back starts to arch off the floor or the abs begin to quiver, you are putting a strain on the back. **Try again with the leg higher, but if you still feel any discomfort stop immediately.**

3. Take another long full breath and, as you breathe out, change the legs so the second leg is drawn in towards the chest and the first is stretched out. Always keep the whole back on the floor. Alternate 5–10 times on each side.

Variation

When you can do this exercise with ease, try it with your head raised, curling towards the knees. This makes the exercise a lot more difficult and, if you feel a strain in the neck or shoulders, release back down to the floor.

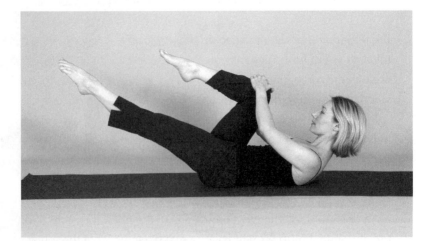

The Cobra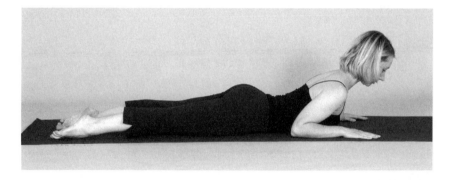

This is not the same as the yoga Cobra exercise – you do not arch the spine to look up at the ceiling. However, it is a powerful, strengthening exercise for the abdominal and lower buttock muscles.

1. Lie face down on the floor with the feet slightly apart and the hands level with the head, palms and elbows on the floor. Breathe in and, as you breathe out, draw the navel to the spine and engage the muscles in the lowest part of the buttocks and the pelvic floor.

2. Draw the shoulders and the muscles of the upper back down and at the same time lift the head off the floor, keeping the chest open. Keep the head in line with the spine – don't try to look up to the ceiling – and put as little pressure as possible on your hands and arms.

3. Breathe in to return to the starting position. Repeat up to 10 times.

Inner Thigh Lifts

This exercise tones the often neglected muscles along the inner thigh.
Rest your back against a wall to ensure you are in alignment.

1. Lie on your side, with your back flat against the wall, the lower leg
   stretched out in line with your back. Bend your upper leg so that the
   knee forms a right angle and place the knee on a cushion. Rest your
   head on your lower arm and place the other hand in front of you for
   support.

2. Breathe in and, as you breathe out, draw the navel to the spine and
   lift the lower leg, keeping the foot extended forwards. The effort
   should all take place in the thigh and abdominal muscles. If you feel
   tension in the upper body, take the leg lower.

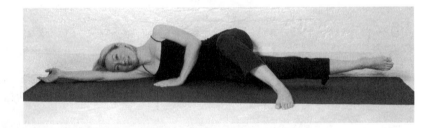

3. Lower and repeat up to 10 times on each leg.

Variation

*If you find this exercise easy, try it with a flexed foot and, to make it
harder still, add a 2lb, or 1kg, ankle weight.*

Arm Toning and Stretching

This sequence tones and strengthens the arms, ending in a stretch to release the muscles. For maximum effort, use weights (2 lb, or 1kg weights are ideal) or improvise with food cans! Most importantly, though, feel when your arms are moving that the movement starts from the middle of the back, and the shoulders and neck are free from tension.

1. Stand about a foot away from a wall, with your feet hip-width apart. Bend the knees a little and lean back against the wall so that the entire length of the spine is in contact with the wall. You will need to draw the navel back towards the spine for this.

2. Breathe in and, as you breathe out, keep the navel drawn towards the spine. Draw down your shoulder blades as you raise your arms straight out to the sides. Bring them as far as you can towards shoulder height without lifting the shoulders or tensing the neck. Repeat 10 times.

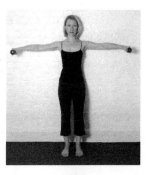

3. Check your posture and now lift your arms 10 times to the front, bending at the elbows to raise your hands to your shoulders. Again, be sure to keep the shoulders dropped and relaxed.

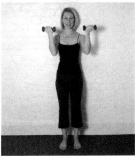

Windmill Arms

This is a good exercise for releasing tension and mobilizing the shoulders. Don't try to force the arms to go beyond their natural limit or you will distort the spine.

1. Lie with your knees raised and your feet flat on the floor. Feel your back release along the floor and then, without losing that feeling, raise your arms so that the fingertips point up to the ceiling.

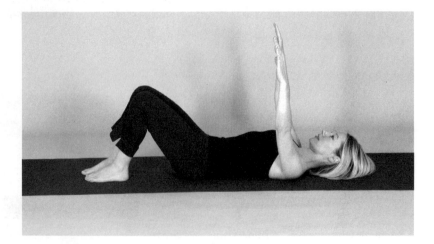

2. Breathe in and, as you breathe out, draw the navel to the spine and take the arms in opposite directions – one above your head, palm up, the other down by your side, palm down. If the arm behind your head does not reach the floor, don't worry – just take it as far as it will go without straining.

3. Rotate the arms as you breathe in until the arms have reversed their positions, so that your first arm is by your side, the second above your head.

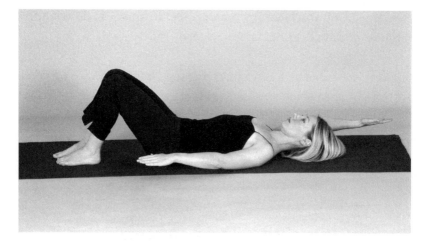

4. As you breathe out, lift the arms up and repeat the sequence for up to 10 times.

Cat With a Leg Stretch

This is a variation on the Cat exercise that you learned during pregnancy (*see page* 66). **If you have any back problems, however, do not attempt this one: stick to the original Cat instead.**

1. Kneel down on all fours, elongating your spine and keeping your neck in line with it. You are aiming at a completely flat, table-top back! Make sure there is no tension in the neck or shoulders.

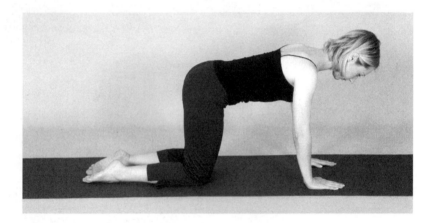

2. Breathe in and, as you breathe out, draw the navel to the spine and raise the right knee up towards the chest, dropping your head down to meet it.

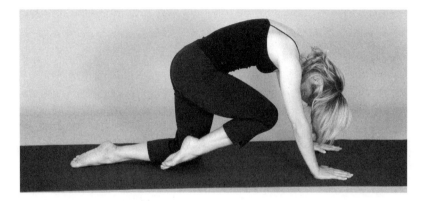

3. Breathe in and straighten the leg out behind you, raising the head back to the starting position. Repeat up to 10 times with each leg.

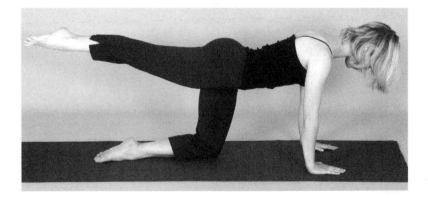

Dog Pose

After the cat – the dog! This is a lovely stretch to do after the last exercise, releasing any tension that may have crept in to the back or neck.

1. Begin in the same position as the last exercise, then tuck your toes under, breathing out and drawing the navel to the spine. Now, press up from the floor so that the soles of your feet are flat and you make a triangle, with your bottom as the apex. Straighten your legs as much as possible, keeping your back long, the head and neck in line with the spine. Try to extend the stretch as you take long, deep breaths, checking that there is no tension in the neck or shoulders. Hold for up to a minute.

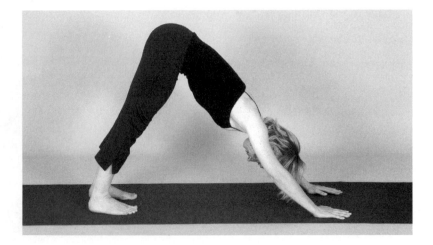

2. Drop your knees back down to the floor and then sit back on your heels with your arms stretched out in front of you – the Child's Pose (page 83). Rest your head on the floor, on one side if that is more comfortable. Relax into this position and breathe deeply.

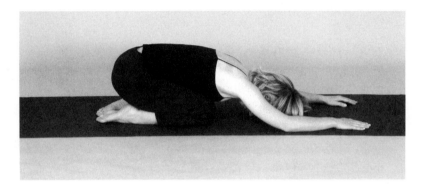

Ankle Circles

This is more than just an ankle exercise. It tones up the thighs and buttocks, too. It is important to sit very tall throughout this – if you find it difficult, sit with your back against a wall.

1. Sit on the floor with your legs straight out in front of you. Feel your body pulled up away from the floor with a long spine. Engage the buttock muscles so you are up on your 'sitting bones'. Draw the navel to the spine, check that the shoulders and neck are relaxed and place your hands in front of your body. Point the toes.

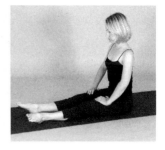

2. Flex the feet back hard so that your toes and knees are pointing up at the ceiling. Your heels may come off the floor. Slowly turn the feet out into a V-shape, but feel the movement begin, not at the ankles, but in the thighs and buttocks.

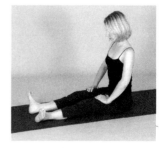

3. Keeping the turn-out, point the feet and return to the starting position. Repeat up to 10 times.

Leg Toning with Weights

This is the same as the exercise from second trimester of pregnancy (*see page* 63), but with the addition of 2lb, or 1kg, ankle weights.

Squeeze

Follow the last exercise with the Cushion Squeeze, page 68.

Relaxation Sequence

Finish your exercise session with the Relaxation Sequence given on page 45.

10

Six Months Plus

The exercises in this section are going to tone and define your body and are a lot more strenuous than the ones you have been doing so far. Don't move on to them just because you have reached the six-month mark after the birth of your baby. Only progress on to these if you can do all of the previous section comfortably and introduce them gradually into your routine as you get stronger. Start with the Warm-up (page 23) followed by the exercises from the previous section and incorporate the following new exercises as and when you feel ready.

Sit-ups PELVIC FLOOR

You can now start to really strengthen your abdominal muscles. Take it slowly at first, though, or you may find the effort is in your back rather than your abs – and that will not only defeat the object, but it will give you back problems as well. Always prepare as you did for the Pelvic Tilt (page 116), engaging the abdominal and low buttock muscles. And, if you feel any strain in the back, or if your abdominal muscles quiver or bulge out with the effort, it means you have come up too far, so take it lower until you feel stronger.

1. Lie on your back with your knees raised and your feet flat on the floor. Place a cushion or a rolled-up towel between your knees to remind you to keep your legs still and check there is no tension in your neck or shoulders. Place your hands lightly behind your head – don't use them to hoist yourself up during the exercise.

2. Breathe in and, as you breathe out, draw the navel to the spine; engage the pelvic floor and low buttock muscles and start to curl your head and shoulders off the floor. If you can only raise your head to start with, don't worry – just keep working at this level until you are stronger. The most important thing to check is that your abs are not bulging or quivering with the effort. If they are, don't lift your head and shoulders so far off the floor. Another sign you have come too far off the floor is if the neck and shoulders start to tense. The neck should be long, the shoulders down and you should be looking ahead, rather than down to your body.

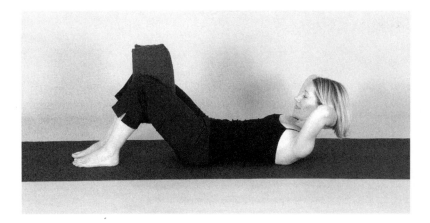

3. When you have come up as far as you can without straining, breathe in and roll down to the floor. Check for tension, especially in the upper body or the jaw. Rest if you need to and then repeat up to 10 times.

Oblique Sit-ups

This exercise also strengthens the abdominal muscles, but this time it is those at the sides of the body. As in the previous exercise, **curl up only as far as you can without feeling the strain in your back or neck.**

1. Lie on your back, as in the previous exercise with your hands held lightly behind your head. Keep your shoulders and neck relaxed.

2. Breathe in and, as you breathe out, draw the navel to the spine, engage the low buttock muscles and curl up to bring your left shoulder in the direction of your right knee. As in the previous exercise, if the abdominal muscles start to bulge or quiver, if there is any strain in the back or tension in the neck or shoulders, you are coming up too far from the floor.

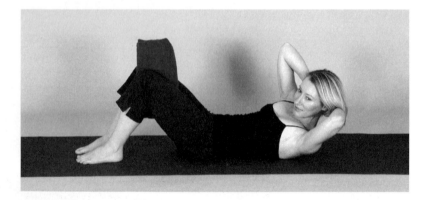

3. Breathe in and lower to the floor. Repeat up to 5 times on each side.

Advanced Pelvic Tilts Sequence

This exercise combines pelvic tilts with sit-ups. If you feel any strain doing sit-ups, stop at Step 5. It is a good idea before you start this exercise to do some pelvic tilts as a warm-up to mobilize the back (*see page* 116).

1. Lie on your back, knees raised with a cushion between them, feet flat on the floor. Check that there is no tension in the neck or shoulders and feel the spine long and flat against the floor.

2. Breathe in and, as you breathe out, draw the navel to the spine, engaging the pelvic floor and low buttock muscles. Start to scoop out the abdomen and curl the spine up from the floor, vertebra by vertebra. Aim for a diagonal shape – don't push up too far or you will arch the back.

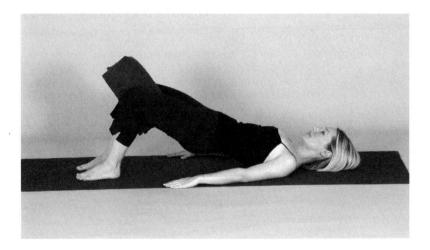

3. Holding your body in this diagonal shape – this requires some effort on the part of your abdominal muscles – and checking there is no tension in the neck or shoulders, breathe in and raise your arms, lifting them above your head and, if you can, placing them on the floor behind your head.

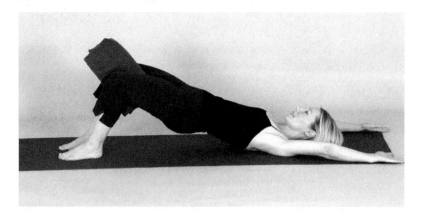

4. Keeping your arms behind you, breathe out and curl the spine back down to the floor vertebra by vertebra, making it as long and straight as you can. You will feel a strong stretch in the arms.

5. Breathe in and make a wide circle with your arms on the floor back down towards your side. If you are confident you are strong enough to include a sit-up, go on to Step 6. If not, repeat the steps so far up to 10 times.

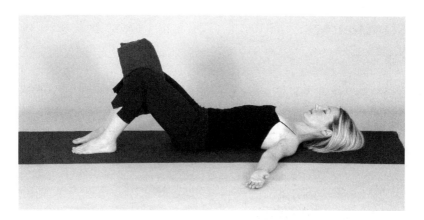

6. Lift your arms so they are off the floor, parallel to your body, the fingertips pointing towards your feet. As you breathe out, draw the navel to the spine and, keeping the neck and shoulders free from tension, curl the head and shoulders off the floor.

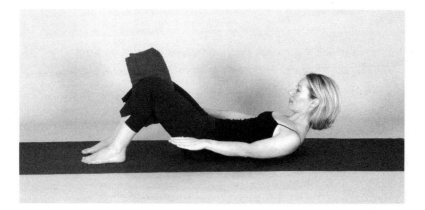

7. Breathe in and lower slowly back to the floor. Repeat the whole sequence up to 10 times.

Star Stretches PELVIC FLOOR

This exercise strengthens the abdominal, gluteal and back muscles. It is important to keep the navel drawn well into the spine all the way through to protect the back. Place a small cushion under your abdomen to remind you to keep those muscles well pulled up.

1. Lie on the floor on your front with a small cushion under the navel, your feet a hip-width apart, the legs and toes stretching away. Stretch your arms above your head, palms down on the floor, but keep the shoulders pulled well down into the back. If you find it more comfortable, place a small cushion or flat towel underneath the forehead.

2. Breathe in and, as you breathe out, draw the navel well up towards the spine, pull up the pelvic floor muscles and maintain this throughout the exercise. On the next out-breath, stretch your right arm and left leg so that they lift two inches off the floor.

3. Breathe in to return to the starting position and, on the next out-breath, lift the left arm and right leg. Repeat up to 5 times on each side.

4. If you are strong enough, now try to lift both arms and both legs on the next out-breath. If this movement distorts your pelvis or back, however, just practise the previous stages.

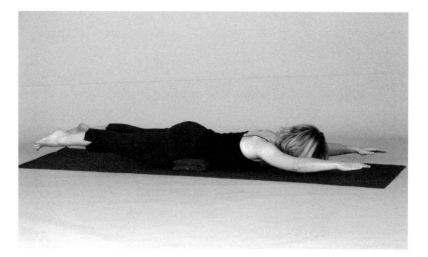

5. Repeat up to 5 times, and then rest in the Child's Pose (*see page* 83).

Side Stretches

This is a stronger movement than it looks as you are lifting the weight of both legs. It is important to lift them only as far as they will go without distorting the back or pelvis, or tensing up the shoulders and neck.

1. Lie on your side with your back against a wall, your legs stretched out in line with your back. Place your lower arm on the floor and rest your head on it, with your upper arm on the floor in front of you as support. Your face, shoulders, hips and knees should all be facing directly forwards. Check there is no tension in the neck or shoulders.

2. Breathe in and, as you breathe out, draw the navel to the spine, flex the feet and lift them two or three inches off the floor. Stretch away with the heels rather than lifting the legs high. Take care not to let the hips roll or the back come away from the wall.

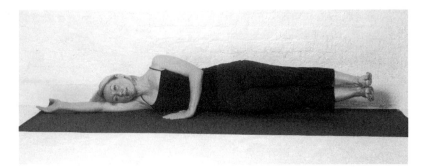

3. Breathe in to lower the legs. Check there is no tension in the shoulders or neck and repeat up to 10 times.

Tricep Dips

This is a very effective arm toning exercise. You use your own body weight as resistance. Make sure the chair you use is heavy and cannot tip up.

1. Sit on a chair with your knees and feet together, back straight and your hands holding on to the edge of the seat. Check you have no tension in the shoulders or neck and the shoulders are dropped down into the back.

2. Breathe in and, as you breathe out, draw the navel to the spine and move off the edge of the chair, still in the same seated position but with nothing underneath you. Let your bottom drop down a few inches, supporting your back with your arms.

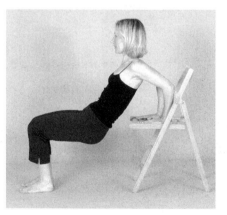

3. Breathe out and rise up a few inches. Repeat up to 10 times.

The Hundred

This is one of the best-known Pilates exercises and very strenuous it is, too, especially on the abdominal muscles! Work up to it slowly and only after you are comfortable with sit-ups. If you start to tense up the shoulders or neck, or feel any strain in the back, stop immediately.

1. Lie on your back and draw your knees up so that your thighs form a right angle to your chest, keeping them parallel and your feet pointed. Your arms are stretched out, with pointed fingers, just a few inches from your sides.

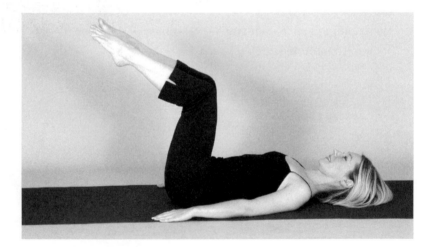

2. Breathe in and, as you breathe out, draw the navel to the spine and lift your head to look straight towards your thighs and lift your arms a few inches off the floor. Tap your hands on to the floor 5 times.

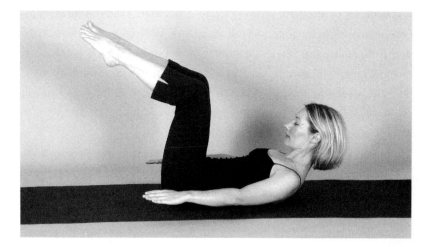

3. Breathe in, keeping the navel drawn to the spine, and make another 5 taps. Repeat, 5 times on each in-breath, 5 times on each out-breath, working up over time until you have reached 100 taps. If you feel tension at any time, lower down to the ground and relax. However many taps you reach, always finish the exercise by lowering the head to the ground and hugging the knees to the chest for a few moments.

Double Leg Stretch PELVIC FLOOR

This is a simplified version of another classic Pilates exercise and, again, it takes a lot of strength, so work up to it gradually, beginning with just one or two repetitions and trying these only when you are comfortable with sit-ups and the single leg stretch. Don't do this one if you have neck or back problems and, if you feel a strain in the neck or back at any time, lower the head back down to the floor and hug the knees in to the chest.

1. Lie on your back and bend the knees up to your chest so the knees are apart and the toes are together, your hands resting just below your knees. Breathe in and, as you breathe out, draw the navel to the spine, pull up the pelvic floor muscles and, without tensing the neck or shoulders, curl the head off the floor so you are looking towards your knees.

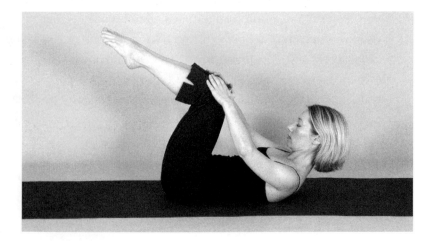

2. Breathe in and, as you breathe out, still firmly holding on to the abdominal muscles, straighten the legs upwards and reach out with the arms so that they are parallel to the body, with pointed fingers.

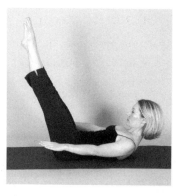

3. As you breathe in, turn out the legs from the hip sockets and flex the feet – this will extend the stretch in the legs.

4. Breathe out and bring the arms up towards your face, behind your head and in a wide circle back to where they started.

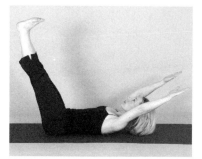 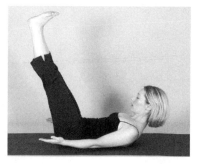

5. Breathe in and lower your head to the floor and bend the knees to bring the legs to their starting position. Relax for a moment. Over time, as you get stronger, repeat this exercise, working up to 10 times.

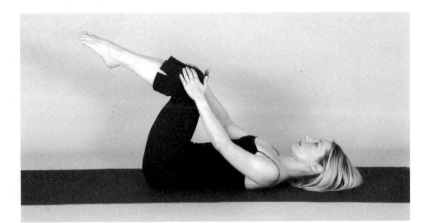

Roll Downs with a Swing

After all that tough abdominal work, it's time to loosen out the muscles. This exercise is one long, continuous ripple of the body.

If at any time you feel dizzy during this exercise, stop immediately.

1. Stand with your feet a hip-width apart, your back straight and your shoulders relaxed. Lift both arms up above your head, slightly in front of your body, with the palms facing you. Bend your knees and begin to curl down, letting your back arch, and keeping your gaze directed at your palms. Let your arms bend, too.

2. When you have bent your knees as far as they will go without the heels coming off the floor, look down to the floor and let your body roll down onto your knees.

3. As soon as your chest makes contact with your thighs, start to straighten your legs as far as they will go without straining; let your body hang upside down from the waist like a rag doll, with no tension in the neck or shoulders.

4. Continue the movement as you start to uncurl slowly to a standing position, bringing your spine up, vertebra by vertebra, to a tall, elongated line. Your neck and head are the last to uncurl. Lift the arms and repeat 4 times.

5. Repeat the previous stages but this time let your arms swing behind you naturally, feeling loose in the shoulder sockets, as you curl down. Repeat 4 times.

Side Stretches with Arms

Now that your spine is feeling more supple, this exercise stretches you out sideways. It is important to keep the hips and the whole upper body facing directly forwards throughout.

1. Stand with the feet hip-width apart and slightly turned out, with a long, straight back and relaxed shoulders. Breathe in and, as you breathe out, draw the navel to the spine and lift up out of the waist.

2. Let your right hand start to slide down your right leg, trying to retain the feeling of lift in the ribs. Reach as far as you can, feeling the stretch up the left side of the body and taking care to keep facing square to the front.

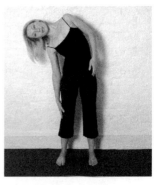

3. Breathe in and, as you breathe out, come up and repeat 5 times on each side.

Variation

When you can do the previous exercise easily, you can extend the stretch by using the opposite arm.

1. Stand as before, this time with your right hand on your waist. Breathe in and, as you breathe out, draw the navel to the spine and lift up out of the waist. Raise your left arm above your head.

2. Bend the upper body to the right as before, taking your left arm with you, stretching out beyond your head. Keep your upper arm close to the side of your face and take care to keep facing square to the front.

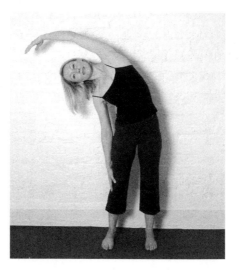

3. Breathe in and, as you breathe out, return to the starting position. Repeat up to 5 times on each side.

Wide Leg Circles

This is really two exercises rolled into one that both stretches and tones the legs and the abs. Make sure the effort is in the abdominal muscles and the legs and keep the upper body – particularly the shoulders and neck – relaxed.

1. Lie on your back with your legs stretched out, parallel, with the knees facing the ceiling and toes pointed. Check that your shoulders are drawn down into your back and your arms are relaxed at your side. Breathe in and, as you breathe out, draw the navel to the spine and hold this position throughout the exercise.

2. Take another in-breath and, keeping the navel held to the spine, raise the left leg to the ceiling and, if you are flexible, towards your body. Keep your leg straight and the toe pointed. If your back comes off the floor or starts to feel a strain, stop immediately.

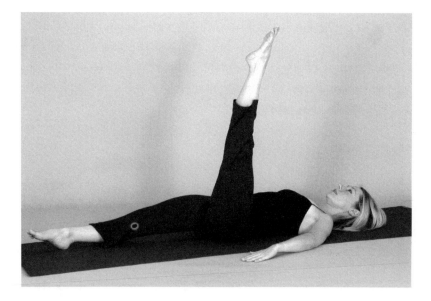

3. Lower the leg and repeat up to 5 times on each side. Relax for a few moments and, if you feel strong enough, go on to the next step.

4. Raise your arms up to shoulder height but keep them relaxed on the floor. Breathe in and, as you breathe out, draw the navel to the spine and keep it held there throughout the rest of the exercise.

5. Keeping it on the floor, move your left leg out to the side, as if you were tracing a circle with your toes. Inevitably, you will have to lift the leg off the floor at some point, but continue to keep it as low as you can while you continue with the circle.

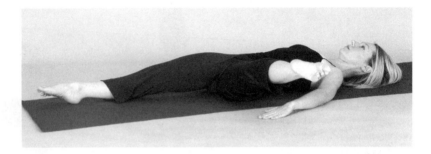

6. When the leg has reached as far as it can, take it over the body, still keeping the circle as wide as possible. Let the leg continue its circle down the other side of your body, keeping as much as possible of your back on the floor, especially your shoulders. Continue until the leg crosses back to the starting position. Repeat, alternating the legs, twice on each side.

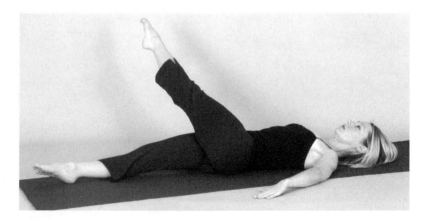

The Bridge

The bridge both mobilizes and strengthens the back. **Do not do this one if you have a back problem. Always stop if you feel a strain.**

1. Lie on your back with your knees raised, heels close to your bottom, arms by your sides. Your back should be in a long straight line all the way through to your neck. Draw your navel to your spine and tilt your chin downwards slightly, for maximum lengthening of the spine. Make sure there is no tension in the shoulders or neck.

2. Breathe in and, as you breathe out, lengthen the back even more, relaxing your upper body. On the next out-breath, begin to curl up from the floor, starting with the buttocks and working up, vertebra by vertebra through the spine. If you can, come all the way up to your shoulders, then hold for a few moments, breathing normally.

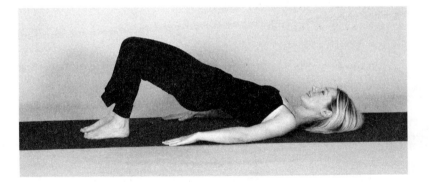

3. On the next out-breath, curl back down so that your buttocks are the last part to touch the floor. Repeat, slowly, up to 5 times.

Sitting Forward Stretch

This exercise stretches and releases the back muscles in the opposite direction from the previous exercise.

1. Sit up with a long straight spine and your legs in front of you on the floor, knees facing the ceiling and toes pointed. Relax the upper body, draw the navel to the spine and engage the buttock muscles – you should grow taller by about two inches!

2. Breathe in and, as you breathe out, hinge in the hip sockets so that you reach forwards over your legs, the top of your head leading the way. Try not to let the shoulders tense up or the back round. This is a long, slow stretch and it's better to keep the length in the back rather than try to get as low as possible.

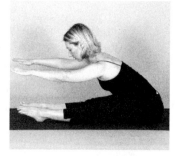

3. On the next out-breath, try to release the lower back more so that you reach a little further. Repeat over the next four or five out-breaths, each time taking the stretch a little further.

Shoulder Release

This is an excellent way of releasing tension in the shoulders, but don't strain to get your fingers clasped as that will undo any possible benefit. Instead use a scarf or belt and the shoulders will loosen over time. You will probably find one side is much looser than the other.

1. Kneel down so that you are sitting on your heels with a long, straight back. Breathe in and, as you breathe out, draw your navel to your spine and release any tension in the shoulders and neck.

2. Take your scarf or belt in your right hand and stretch the right arm up to the ceiling, then bend it at the elbow so the right hand reaches down behind your neck, the scarf or belt hanging down your back.

3. Reach your left arm behind your back so that the left hand catches hold of the scarf or belt as close as it can to the right hand. Hold this position for several long, slow breaths, trying to release the shoulders more. If you can touch the fingers of your two hands easily, you can dispense with the scarf or belt and simply clasp the fingers together. Repeat on the other side.

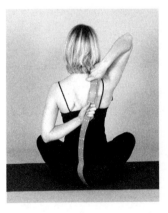

Cushion Squeeze

Follow this with the Cushion Squeeze exercise, as on page 68.

Relaxation Sequence

Finish your exercise session, as always, with the Relaxation Sequence on page 45.

Index

digestive system 12
Dog pose 126–7
double leg stretch 144–6

E

endorphins 10
exercise 12–14

F

feet
    arching 73
    exercise 107
    massage 74
    pointing/flexing 90–1
    standing posture 18
first three months post-pregnancy
    89–108
first trimester
    exercise regime 27–49
    guidelines 12–13
    standing posture 17–18
flowing movements 8
fluid retention 11, 71, 92
forward bend 41–2

G

girdle of strength 7, 18, 25
    foot exercise 107
    pelvic floor 101, 102
    standing side stretch 103
gluteal stretch 115
Graham, Martha 2

H

haemorrhoids 11, 27, 28
hamstrings
    sitting with legs apart 81
    spinal twist 80
    stretches 114
hand exercise 76
head
    rolls 33–4, 89
    standing posture 17
    tilts 33–4, 89
heart rate 10
heartburn 12, 71
heel lifts 100
hips
    rolls 57
    sitting with legs apart 81
    squatting 65
    turn-out 106

NATURAL WELL WOMAN

A Practical Guide to Health and Wellbeing for Life

Dr Penny Stanway

Compiled by a highly regarded women's health specialist, *Natural Well Woman* is a full colour, totally comprehensive guide to health and wellbeing. It is informative and relevant to women of all ages.

Taking into account the changing needs during each stage of life, *Natural Well Woman* provides simple, authoritative advice and insights into health matters and natural health, including:

- The definitive guide to staying fit
- Healthy advice about dieting and nutrition
- Guidance for relationships, stress management, relaxation and spiritual health
- An authoritative overview of complementary and alternative health treatments
- A comprehensive index of symptoms and treatment for common ailments

Dr Penny Stanway is a respected authority on women's health. She writes and lectures on a range of issues - in particular pregnancy, breastfeeding and natural health. She is a columnist for *Women's Weekly* magazine and was the co-author (with husband Dr Andrew Stanway) of the classic bestseller *Breast Is Best.*

ISBN 1-86204-791-X

Order now at www.thorsons.com

COMPLETE WOMEN'S HEALTH

The Essential and Comprehensive Health Companion for Every Stage of Your Life

The Royal College of Obstetricians and Gynaecologists

A complete reference book for every phase of a woman's life – from puberty, to pregnancy, menopause and old age.

Complete Women's Health is packed with factual, helpful information on health care for women of all ages. Compiled by a team of leading doctors and medical experts, it is the ultimate guide to women's health, written in a user-friendly, non-technical language. This practical, illustrated manual will help women to:

- Take preventative action to protect and preserve their health
- Respond quickly and appropriately to symptoms that occur
- Know what questions to ask their doctor or specialist

Subjects covered include: heavy and painful periods, PMS, pregnancy and childbirth, miscarriage, infertility, menopause, hysterectomy, osteoporosis, heart health, sexual health and contraception, women's cancers and gynaecological problems.

ISBN 0-7225-3430-2   **Order now at www.thorsons.com**

PREPARING FOR BIRTH WITH YOGA

Empowering and Effective Exercise for Pregnancy and Childbirth

Janet Balaskas

This book adopts an approach to yoga that is designed to help the expectant mother to develop confidence in her body. Avoiding complicated jargon, it explains in detail how to attune to natural energies and how an understanding of gravity can be used beneficially during pregnancy and birth. The illustrated exercises show how yoga can strengthen the body, help it to become more supple, and relieve stress.

Janet Balaskas is the founder of the Active Birth Movement.

ISBN 1-85230-431-6   **Order now at www.thorsons.com**

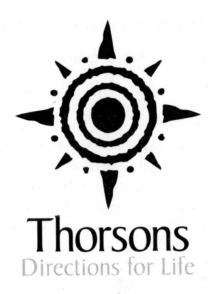

Thorsons
Directions for Life

This online sanctuary is packed with information, inspiration and guidance to help you on the path to physical and spiritual well-being. Drawing on the integrity and vision of our authors and titles, and with health advice, articles, astrology, tarot, a meditation zone, author interviews and events listings, Thorsons.com is a great alternative to help create space and peace in our lives.

So if you've always wondered about practising yoga, following an allergy-free diet, using the tarot or getting a life coach, we can point you in the right direction.

Make www.thorsons.com your online sanctuary.

www.thorsons.com